WHEN THE BODY SPEAKS

WHEN THE BODY SPEAKS
Psychological Meanings in Kinetic Clues

---

edited by
Selma Kramer, M.D., and
Salman Akhtar, M.D.

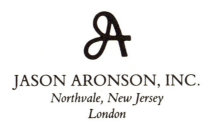

JASON ARONSON, INC.
Northvale, New Jersey
London

Copyright © 1992 by Jason Aronson Inc.

10 9 8 7 6 5 4 3 2 1

All rights reserved. Printed in the United States of America. No part of this book may be used or reproduced in any manner whatsoever without written permission from Jason Aronson Inc. except in the case of brief quotations in reviews for inclusion in a magazine, newspaper, or broadcast.

Production Editors: Gloria Jordan and Leslie Block
Editorial Director: Muriel Jorgensen
This book was set in 11½/14 Bem by Lind Graphics, Upper Saddle River, NJ, and printed and bound by Haddon Craftsmen, Scranton, PA.

Library of Congress Cataloging-in-Publication Data

When the body speaks : psychological meanings in kinetic clues /
  edited by Selma Kramer and Salman Akhtar.
     p. cm.
  "Originally presented at the Twenty-second Annual Margaret S. Mahler Symposium on Child Development held on May 18, 1991, in Philadelphia"—Acknowledgments.
  Includes bibliographical references and index.
  ISBN 0-87668-461-4
  1. Nonverbal communication (Psychology)—Congresses.
  2. Psychoanalytic interpretation—Congresses. 3. Separation
-individuation—Congresses. I. Kramer, Selma. II. Akhtar, Salman,
  1946 July 31-   III. Margaret S. Mahler Symposium on Child
Development (22nd : 1991 : Philadelphia, Pa.)
  [DNLM: 1. Nonverbal Communication—congresses. 2. Psychoanalytic
Interpretation—congresses. WM 460.5.C5 W567 1991]
  RC489.N65W54   1992
  616.89'17—dc20
DNLM/DLC
for Library of Congress   91-45288

Manufactured in the United States of America. Jason Aronson Inc. offers books and cassettes. For information and catalog, write to Jason Aronson Inc., 230 Livingston Street, Northvale, New Jersey 07647.

*To the memory of
Margaret S. Mahler—
teacher, friend, source of inspiration*

Contents

Acknowledgment　　　　　　　　　　xi

Contributors　　　　　　　　　　　xiii

1
Nonverbal Manifestations of Unresolved Separation-Individuation in Adult Psychopathology　　1
Selma Kramer, M.D.

2
Tethers, Orbits, and Invisible Fences: Clinical, Developmental, Sociocultural, and Technical Aspects of Optimal Distance　　21
Salman Akhtar, M.D.

3
Vicissitudes of Optimal Distance Through the Life Cycle   59
Discussion of Akhtar's Chapter, "Tethers, Orbits, and Invisible Fences: Clinical, Developmental, Sociocultural, and Technical Aspects of Optimal Distance"
Philip J. Escoll, M.D.

4
A Problem with the Couch: Incapacities and Conflicts   89
Alvin Frank, M.D.

5
Unresolved Separation-Individuation, Masochism, and Difficulty with Compliance   113
Discussion of Frank's Chapter, "A Problem With The Couch: Incapacities and Conflicts"
LeRoy J. Byerly, M.D.

6
Nonverbal Behaviors in the Analytic Situation: The Search for Meaning in Nonverbal Cues   131
James T. McLaughlin, M.D.

7
Gestures, Emblems, and Body Language: What Does It All Mean?   163
Discussion of McLaughlin's Chapter "Nonverbal Behaviors in the Analytic Situation: The Search for Meaning in Nonverbal Cues"
Sydney E. Pulver, M.D.

8
Technical Applications of the Nonverbal Aspects of Separation-Individuation Phenomena 179
A Concluding Commentary on Akhtar's, Frank's, and McLaughlin's Chapters
Bernard L. Pacella, M.D.

Index 201

Acknowledgment

The chapters in this book were originally presented at the Twenty-Second Annual Margaret S. Mahler Symposium on Child Development held on May 18, 1991, in Philadelphia. First and foremost, therefore, we wish to express our gratitude to the Margaret S. Mahler Psychiatric Research Foundation. James McLaughlin, M.D., permitted us to use a part of his chapter's title, in slightly modified form, as the subtitle of our book. We thank him for his generosity. We are also grateful to Troy L. Thompson II, M.D., chairman, Department of Psychiatry and Human Behavior, Jefferson Medical College, as well as to the Philadelphia Psychoanalytic Institute and Society for their shared sponsorship of this symposium. Many colleagues from the Institute and Society helped during the symposium, and we remain grateful to them. Finally, we thank Ms. Gloria Schwartz for her efficient organizational assistance during the symposium and outstanding skills in the preparation of this book.

Contributors

Salman Akhtar, M.D.
Professor of Psychiatry, Jefferson Medical College; Faculty, Philadelphia Psychoanalytic Institute, Philadelphia, Pennsylvania.

LeRoy J. Byerly, M.D.
Training and Supervising Analyst, Philadelphia Psychoanalytic Institute, Philadelphia, Pennsylvania.

Philip J. Escoll, M.D.
Training and Supervising Analyst, Philadelphia Psychoanalytic Institute; Clinical Professor of Psychiatry, University of Pennsylvania School of Medicine; Senior Attending Psychiatrist, Institute of Pennsylvania Hospital, Philadelphia, Pennsylvania.

Alvin Frank, M.D.
Training and Supervising Analyst, St. Louis Psychoanalytic Institute; Chairman, Committee on Scientific Activities, American

Psychoanalytic Association; Professor of Clinical Psychiatry, St. Louis University, St. Louis, Missouri.

Selma Kramer, M.D.
Professor of Psychiatry, Jefferson Medical College; Training and Supervising Analyst, Philadelphia Psychoanalytic Institute, Philadelphia, Pennsylvania.

James T. McLaughlin, M.D.
Training and Supervising Analyst, and Former Director, Pittsburgh Psychoanalytic Institute; Associate Clinical Professor Emeritus of Psychiatry, School of Medicine, University of Pittsburgh, Pittsburgh, Pennsylvania.

Bernard L. Pacella, M.D.
President, American Psychoanalytic Association; Clinical Professor Emeritus of Psychiatry, College of Physicians and Surgeons, Columbia University; Faculty, Columbia Psychoanalytic Institute; Member, New York Psychoanalytic Institute, New York.

Sydney E. Pulver, M.D.
Training and Supervising Analyst, Philadelphia Psychoanalytic Institute; Clinical Professor of Psychiatry, University of Pennsylvania School of Medicine. Philadelphia, Pennsylvania.

1

NONVERBAL MANIFESTATIONS OF UNRESOLVED SEPARATION-INDIVIDUATION IN ADULT PSYCHOPATHOLOGY

Selma Kramer, M.D.

> I would be even more emphatic now about the need to pay attention to nonverbal communication . . . than I have been in years past. The psychoanalytic situation stresses the importance of speech in contrast to action. The analysand's position on the couch, by subtle suggestion, limits the extent of active movement, and the suggestion is furthered by the direction to the analysand to speak whatever thoughts and feelings he becomes aware of during the hour. Yet the movements on the couch, postures, mannerisms, changes in tone and intensity of voice, flushing, sweating, and special states of body tension are all part of the expression of feeling and may represent explicit communications. [Greenacre 1971, pp. 61–62]

These words of Phyllis Greenacre, a highly esteemed colleague of Margaret Mahler, not only remind us of the significance of the nonverbal communications of our patients but also set the stage for my own contribution here. In this chapter I undertake an exploration of the nonverbal elements in the analytic situation and their possible links to the symbiotic phase of development and the subsequent separation–individuation process. I begin with a brief review of the body's role in symbiosis and the separation–individuation phase, frequently illustrating my points with brief clinical vignettes. Following this, I present an analytic case where "decoding" certain nonverbal communications led to a deeper understanding of the patient's problems and their amelioration. This leads to the last section of the chapter, in which I discuss certain technical matters specific to child analysis and the impact of such conceptualization on working with adults.

SYMBIOSIS AND SEPARATION–INDIVIDUATION: THE ROLE OF THE BODY

Symbiosis

The distinctive characteristics of each infant are themselves the result of

> the interaction between the infant's equipment and early experiential factors—an interaction that aggravates or attenuates initial tendencies—[which] will lean, after a few weeks, to the emergence of basic core of fundamental trends with which the infant enters the symbiotic phase. [Weil 1970, p. 402]

In the symbiotic phase, as far as the child is concerned, there is no separateness between himself and mother. They are together enveloped, as it were, by a common shell. What touches him, pains him, comforts him, is felt to arise from within for, at this time, the child is directed proprioceptively. Mahler's work with psychotic and ego-impaired children, her analyses of adults, and her observations on normally developing infants led her to these conclusions. While she recognized that there was no method of validating this hypothesis, she felt strongly that it was impossible to accept the opposite hypothesis, namely, that the infant of a few weeks is able to differentiate "self" from "other." Mahler followed Freud's dictum that the ego "is first and foremost a bodily ego" (Freud 1923, p. 26) and acknowledged that orality is in its dominance during symbiosis. In addition, the child's eyes (his looking at and capturing the object's glance by his own) and libidinization of the child's body by the mother's touch play an important role during this developmental stage. These contribute to a gradual shift from mainly proprioenteroceptive to sensoriperceptive experiences.

The significance of both these somatic inputs (i.e., the visual modality and the maternal ministrations) was further investigated by Mahler and her colleagues as well as by other investigators. Mahler and McDevitt (1982), for instance, stated that human infants require boundary sensations conveyed by skin (touch and pain) and by other sensoriperceptive organs, and eventually by motor coordination. In addition to mechanisms of self-boundary formation, the body–self schemata "concerns integration of the body part schemata into a whole body image . . ." (p. 833). The mother's stimulation of the child's body helps form the basis of his later dyadic relationship with her. Indeed, "the sense of self that results will bear the imprint of her caregiving" (p. 837). Riess (1978), studying "the early phases of eye contact between mother and child as one major aspect of their evolving emotional interaction" (p. 382), emphasized the role of vision in development. She felt that the visual feedback between mother and child may leave "visual traces" in the child's personality development, that is, proneness to pleasures, disturbances, or conflicts expressed in the visual mode.

The sequence of frustration followed by gratification slowly gives rise to a budding awareness that there is someone "out there," and to the gradual realization in the infant that he is able to evoke relief through his efforts. Frustrating experiences, therefore, have some constructive influence on the psychic development as well (see also Jacobson 1964 in this regard). This is often not known to (or, for dynamic reasons is overlooked by) parents who, in a misapplication of developmental concepts, vow to never frustrate their child. Many of us have treated children or adolescents raised in this fashion. One such patient was an 11-year-old boy, Aaron, who was failing in school despite the fact that he was very bright. He was friendless, apparently because he did not know how to wait for a turn; he had to be first. The parents' efforts to never frustrate him, to never cause him to cry or even pout, dictated their style of parent–child interaction from the earliest symbiotic phase until the birth of a sibling when Aaron was 3 years old. Aaron's bottle was warmed while he napped so that as soon as he awakened, the nipple was "popped" into his mouth. This "no-frustration" rule was applied to all other aspects of his care; it resulted in a passivity combined with pseudo-omnipotence. This omnipotence was deflated suddenly when the sibling was born. Aaron functioned characterologically as an "exception" (Freud 1916, Jacobson 1959, Kramer 1987), entitled to receive everything without any effort.

Differentiation

In the first few months after birth the sense of touch of and by the infant is of great importance. By 4 months, the baby mouths, touches, and looks at his own fingers.[1] At the same time, there is rapt interest in looking at the mother's face and a growing awareness of the "other than mother." The baby now feels less like a newborn. Although still on the mother's lap (but no longer moulding to her), or at her feet, he looks away from her. It is as though he has a psychic backbone. Libidinization of the body, the desire to see more and more of the surrounding world, and the growth of motor activity promote these early adventures. By

---

1. The use of fingers to soothe or to punish the self is beautifully illustrated in McLaughlin's chapter in this book. Earlier, Hoffer (1952) had emphasized the importance of the baby's touch in becoming familiar with his body's "rind."

3 months of age the nonspecific smile appears, while by 4 to 5 months the smile is specifically for the mother. Sufficient familiarity with the mother's face enables the child to compare her face to that of a stranger. This adds to the recognition, although not yet complete, that he and mother are separate.

An adult male patient in whom differentiation between self and mother was never completed told me on more than one occasion that he had taken aspirin because his mother's arthritis troubled *her*. The patients described by Alvin Frank and James McLaughlin in this book showed the need to keep the analyst in view, a need to see him (and possibly see whether or not he was loving or angry), as well as the possible enactment of an angry rebellion against enforced passivity or against having to lie on the couch (mother's bosom?).

Practicing

Further physical development enables the infant to test and then to practice his motor skills with emotional abandon. With each passing day, this is done at increasing distance from his mother and with such elation that he seems impervious to knocks and bumps. The healthy aggressive endowment of the child impels him to explore the world at large (Parens 1987). At times, his mother's glance, her voice, or her touch are enough to reassure the child by the process known as emotional refueling (Furer, quoted by Mahler 1974, p. 157). The child's growing awareness of the mother's role in setting limits is seen in his teasing of her, as by running into a forbidden area. The mother's response to her child's newfound motility may encourage or dampen his self-confidence and his daring to try new things. The father's role now gains increasing importance and consists of discouraging the mother's overzealous attempts to prevent the child from exercising his autonomy.

Some mothers try to limit the child's explorations by using real or psychic tethers, overcautioning him, as we may surmise from Salman Akhtar's chapter in this book. However, less well known is the fact that where there is too little concern for his safety and whereabouts, the child may construct his own "tether." This may be a result of precocious ego development in a child left to his own devices.

Toward the end of this subphase, cognitive strides as well as the internalization of the mother's protective and soothing style make the child able to comfortably tolerate lengthier separations from his mother. As for physical distance, the child moves farther away.[2] Mahler and McDevitt (1980) emphasize that the stimulating influence of physical prowess "for the establishment of body boundaries and a greater awareness of body parts and body self" (p. 403) is of great importance for identity formation.

Rapprochement

Characteristic of this subphase is the intrapsychic conflict between a desire for fusion with the mother and a strong urge for separateness, individuation, and autonomy. It is manifested physically in the child's alternating approach and distancing behavior, in his darting away from the mother, and in his petulant attempts to coerce her to do his bidding. In her observational research, Mahler felt that this normal intrapsychic conflict was inevitable, regardless of the quality of mothering. This "conflicted" Mahler baby is in contrast to Tolpin's (1980) account of the "happy" Kohut baby (the picture derived from reconstruction, not from observation).

The rapprochement subphase, while tumultuous, is also the most significant insofar as its successful negotiation is accompanied by the following intrapsychic developmental achievements:

---

2. Mahler (personal communication, 1979) alluded to her own need for breaking earlier intellectual and emotional ties when she stated that she could not have conducted her research, or drawn her important conclusions, had she remained in Europe "in the shadows of the titans."

(1) mastery of the cognitively intensified separation anxiety; (2) affirmation of the sense of basic trust; (3) gradual deflation and relinquishment of the sense of omnipotence experienced in the symbiotic dual unity with the mother; (4) gradual compensation for the deflated sense of omnipotence through development of the child's burgeoning ego capacities and sense of autonomy; (5) a firming up of the core sense of self; (6) establishment of a sense of capability for ego control and modulation of strong libidinal and aggressive urges and affects (e.g., infantile rage); (7) healing the developmentally normal tendency to maintain the relation with the love object by splitting it into a "good" and a "bad" object, thus also healing the corresponding intrapsychic split; and (8) supplanting the splitting defense with repression as the later defensive means of curbing unacceptable affects and impulses toward the love object. [Settlage 1977, p. 817]

The good-enough mother promotes the child's physical and emotional steps away by "a benevolent pat on the behind" without herself withdrawing from the child.[3] There are significant differences in how boys and girls negotiate this subphase. First, the boy's greater endowment of aggression enables him to "get out from under" the mother's orbit, while the girl with her "lesser motor-mindedness" (Mahler 1975, p. 214) stays close. Second, while the boy must separate as well as "disidentify" (Greenson 1968) from the mother, the girl has to separate from the mother and at the same time identify with her. Finally, it is during the rapprochement subphase that the girl first becomes aware of her "castrated" state, and compounding her conflict with the mother. As a result of these differences, girls generally show a greater magnitude of rapprochement conflict and more severe rapprochement crises. They are more prone than boys to depressive moods during this subphase.

---

3. It is not an accident, however, that many mothers who cannot tolerate the child's individuation get pregnant again at this time, as if to say "If you do not need me, I will have a baby who does."

Physical manifestation of rapprochement, the ambitendency, with alternating attempts to move away and then to fuse with mother, along with ambivalence (the emotional counterpart of ambitendency), are manifested in the material of all of the authors in this book. Ambitendency is depicted in Akhtar's patients, showing that the fantasy of the tether is not limited to the practicing subphase. A tether fantasy was expressed by my patient Michael, a pseudoindependent 10-year-old boy who insisted on going to overnight camp to get away from his family and from me, none of whom he really needed. He spent the last two weeks before our vacation constructing a very long chain of rubber bands that he fantasied would stretch between us. A yank on the part of either of us would bring the other flying to his side. As an aside, he gloried in the fact that there were no rubber bands for other patients.

Edward, Ruskin, and Turrini (1991) depict another version of a tether in a patient's recollection of a comforting childhood fantasy in which she was a doll and connected to her mother as a puppet is to a puppeteer. I have encountered patients for whom the telephone cord is a tether, at times an intrusive and imperious one. Indeed, the installation of a car phone allowed an agoraphobic patient to leave her home "unaccompanied."

During the rapprochement subphase, growth and development proceed for there are great cognitive strides; speech is well established, and a sense of personal identity and entity are even stronger. By the end of this period, the child's ability to fantasy enables him to soothe himself, to test out increasingly mature roles, and to be more involved with individuals other than mother.

Self and Object Constancy

Reliable and realistic intrapsychic representations of the self and of the primary love objects now enable the child to attain further intrapsychic separation and individuation. Kramer and Akhtar

(1988), in an overview of Mahler's theoretical contributions to psychoanalysis, noted that during this subphase, the child's

> feelings of helplessness and his wish to please his parents while being still angry at them are eased by selective identification with them, leading to increased individuation with sound secondary narcissism and to more complex psychic structure formation. Increasing integration of both self and object representations permits healing of earlier splits between "good" and "bad" self-representations and "good" and "bad" object representations. The child is now tolerant of ambivalence and affectively able to accept both himself and his primary love objects as including good and bad aspects. "Object constancy," or the ability to retain a positively cathected mental representation of the maternal object in her absence and when the child feels ambivalently toward her, is an important achievement of this stage. With the development of "object constancy," and its counterpart "self constancy," the child becomes capable of more complex object relations than were hitherto possible. Increasing disengagement from his first dyadic relationship prepares the child's psyche for the very important triadic form of oedipal relationship. The child is now ready to experience, struggle with, and, one hopes, master newer conflicts. [p. 554]

It is important to note that Mahler referred to this last subphase of the separation as "on the way to self and object constancy," for she felt that object constancy is seldom, if ever, achieved completely. In the early years, by age 3, the average senior toddler is able to tolerate physical separation from his mother in order to attend nursery school. He is able to do this because he has internalized the mothering functions and maintains a well-defined mental representation of her. However, when his body speaks in such a way as to make him unhappy (e.g., when he is ill, hurt, or very tired), the object constancy wears thin. Then the child wants the mother in the flesh.

With the achievement of self and object constancy, there

develops the capacity for triadic oedipal relationships. The interrelationship of the body and intrapsychic processes at this time is well known (Freud 1924, 1925) and does not need restating. Mahler was completely aware of continuities and discontinuities in development. However, she felt strongly that the obligatory precursor to the infantile neurosis, if not its first manifestation, is the rapprochement subphase. The overlapping of the rapprochement with the phallic-oedipal phase interferes with regression "and with the successful passing of the Oedipus complex" (Mahler et al. 1975, p. 227). Mahler emphasized, as did the other members of the 1973 Paris panel, that the shape of the Oedipus complex and the infantile neurosis do not arise anew. Lebovici (1973), Ritvo (1974), Loewald (1974), and Mahler (1975) all agreed that the characterological and neurotic precursors (i.e., the psychic structure forming in the oedipal child) not only create the anlage upon which the Oedipus complex "settles" but determine the fashion in which the sexual drives interact with the state of self and object differentiation and with the self and object relationship reached by the child.

A CLINICAL ILLUSTRATION

In an earlier paper (Kramer and Akhtar 1988) I presented the analysis of a 35-year-old businessman, Mr. G., whom I described as "portly and unkempt." He was chronically depressed. His wife had threatened divorce because of his undue possessiveness, stinginess, and hostility toward their daughter. Mr. G. had been a "replacement child" (Cain and Cain 1964, Poznanski 1972), conceived while his mother was mourning the loss of her father. Throughout his growing up, Mr. G. had felt that he could not be an individual in his own right. He had to live up to his grandfather's intellectual achievements. His self-esteem suffered because he could never seem to match this highly idealized person. Even when he was only 2 years old, family portraits and stories depicted him changing from a clean, well-behaved baby to an angry, stubborn, and physically unclean toddler.

As the dependent and hostile maternal transference developed, Mr. G. came to his sessions increasingly badly dressed, untidy, and smelly. I felt that by doing so he was enacting an early situation that began at age 2 and remained as a character trait as he reached adolescence and adulthood. The establishment of this trait was overdetermined: being sloppy and smelly enabled him to be different from his maternal grandfather, whom he was expected to emulate. It also represented a plea for attention from his depressed mother, who left him in soiled diapers for many hours; at the same time, it was an indictment of her for her neglect.

I knew that his untidiness and his bad body odor were nonverbal communications that had to be treated like any verbal free associations. However, I did not find it easy to confront the patient with what he was doing, for I knew that he was exquisitely sensitive and became hostile or depressed when feeling put down. At the same time, I was not indifferent to the fact that my office reeked during his analytic sessions and for some time thereafter, despite my efforts to deodorize it.

My determination to act (verbally) was abetted by my memory of a paper by Rosen (1964) in which he described his handling of a very smelly, oppositional, and confused adolescent who conceded that "he had been losing respect for me because of my apparent indifference to the odor" (p. 8). I felt that I was being challenged to take a stand with my patient for his sake and for mine, but I knew that he would be unhappy regardless of whether I took the stand and what I said. As I stated in my longer report of this case (Kramer and Akhtar 1988), I felt that

> I would be a bad, rejecting mother if I took note of his slovenliness; I would be the mother who was withdrawn, who ignored him, if I did not. I finally confronted him with the fact that he was demanding my attention to something that would anger him if I

commented on it, namely, the state of his dress and body. He blurted out, "I can come in a tuxedo if you want, but it wouldn't be me." Then, after a long pause he added, "That's the picture of him, the last picture [of his grandfather] before the Nazis came. He wore a full-dress suit because he was being honored." I said, "So, if you come appropriately dressed, you are like your grandfather." He said, "I was beautifully dressed in early pictures; my mother's little prize. I had to play in mud to become myself. Being in mud—what does that mean? My grandfather was shot and left in a ditch by the side of the road. So I'm him no matter what I do!" The split between good and bad self and the pervasive feeling that he could never have his own identity continued to come up for many, many months. [p. 560]

However, after this interchange, Mr. G. gradually became more attentive to his personal hygiene and seemed generally more relaxed with me. I also felt more at ease, no longer having to anticipate his reenactment in the transference of his being a neglected 2-year-old. I believed that he was revealing his identification with the decaying body of his grandfather slain by the Nazis. The smell had been a sort of smoke screen ("smell screen") that had preoccupied both of us.

THE THEORY AND TECHNIQUE OF CHILD ANALYSIS AND THEIR IMPACT ON WORKING WITH ADULTS

Child analysts have somewhat of an advantage over the average adult analyst, for experience convinces us that we must work with nonverbal communications, at times to the exclusion of verbal content.[4] Mahler (1945) said:

---

4. It is noteworthy and exciting that the main chapters of this book and two of the three discussions are written by adult analysts.

> If we are to learn to read the child's emotional language, we are compensated for verbal free association by that very characteristic quality of children tending to betray their *affects* much more directly and immediately than adults. [p. 276, author's emphasis]

Often the child analyst is more active in verbal intervention than is the adult analyst, for he must prepare the child for analytic work by familiarizing him with his mental mechanisms through a process involving running comments, confrontations, and eventually interpretations (Kramer and Byerly 1978). Actually, an important, even a major, difference between child and adult analysis is not in the activity of the analyst but in that of the child. The child is motor-minded and cannot be expected to use the couch except in his play, where he may use it as a trampoline or as a surface on which to enact his fantasies. He cannot verbally free associate. The analyst has the use of the child's sporadic verbal comments but not sustained free associations. He uses the child's nonverbal productions, and especially the child's affects, which are quite transparent in the transference. The analyst must be open to and comfortable with this countertransference.

Some difficulties the child analyst encounters are depicted by Kay (1978) as frustrations that

> form the effects of the domination of the primary process on the child's functioning. The analyst attempts to quickly decipher the child's varied and fluctuating forms of communication, and to respond in an analytically productive way. This requires a unique blend of empathy, dispassionate concern, and insight. . . . [The analyst] must be prepared for the sudden physical exertions or immobility demanded by the child's sudden and frequent changes in mood and behavior. The analyst's position must be maintained in the face of the child's impulsive, provocative behavior and his direct attacks on the analyst's self-esteem. [pp. 317–318]

The countertransference of the child analyst is also more complicated than that of the adult analyst. In addition to the usual triggers for a countertransference reaction experienced by the adult analyst, the child analyst must cope with certain specific factors:

1. There must be a usable relationship, the "informative alliance" (Burlingham 1935), with the parents. This relationship promotes the parents' cooperation during the early phases when the child is uneasy with the procedure, and also when resistances begin to arise in the child. It also counters the fears and resistances of the parents who may withdraw the child from analysis prematurely as soon as there is some symptom improvement or in response to their fears of the analytic process or because of their jealousy of the analyst's importance in the child's life.
2. The child analyst has countertransference responses not only to the material offered by the child but to the child's relationship to his parents as well.
3. Some child analysts may have rescue fantasies based, at least in part, upon their own childhood feelings of deprivation.
4. The child analyst may feel guilty because he is occupied with child patients when he has young children of his own.

What I have described are areas of countertransference that may cause tension in the child analyst, or may actually interfere with his neutrality and openness to complex mental mechanisms. The child analyst with an adequate personal analysis, continuing self-analysis, and confirming experience in the field should be able to work through these potential impediments and use his countertransference in the service of his patient's treatment. It should not be forgotten that, in working with children, it is necessary to distinguish the patient's personal myth (Kris 1956) from the real events of the patient's life.

Aside from the child's physical activity, provocation, and, at times, even personal attacks on the analyst, much of what Kay (1978) has described did occur with the adult patients described by Frank and McLaughlin in their respective chapters. It is obvious that although they had reached chronological maturity, and each consciously came to analysis of his own free will, in many ways the so-called adulthood they were presumed to have reached was a veneer covering pre-oedipal and preverbal issues.[5] These included the deleterious effects of abandonment, loss of primary love objects, helplessness in the face of parental pathology, and illness in the parents. The authors' alertness to the deep pre-oedipal and preverbal issues in adult analyses has given a true technical meaning to "the widening scope of indications for psychoanalysis" (Stone 1954).

The authors lead the readers through the path from pre-oedipal pathology to understand their patients' warped Oedipus complexes. It is important to note that what evolves in the course of an analysis is by no means a carbon copy of the actual events of early life of the infant and toddler. Some authors, criticizing child developmental research and its resultant theories, accuse "developmentalists" of bypassing or minimizing the Oedipus complex. I deny this and agree with Greenacre (personal communication, 1972), who said, "Every patient, with the possible exception of the most severe childhood psychotics, experiences an oedipus, but what an oedipus it is in some!"

Why such a long description of child analysis, and the comparison between adult and child analysis? It is because the enactment in the transference of the patients described by all three major contributors to this volume (Akhtar, Frank, and McLaughlin) are very reminiscent of the "imperativeness and immediacy of the child analytic patient." Mahler (personal com-

---

5. Frank's (1969) remarkable earlier paper, "The Unrememberable and the Unforgettable," also poignantly shows that profound effects of serious preverbal trauma may persist unabated until adulthood.

munication, 1956) once said that "the child analyst may not have the luxury of listening, cogitating, and taking his time to make a comment as does the adult analyst. It is not possible to refrain from verbal or, at times, physical reaction when an anxious child demands help." For the most part, the analysts in the following chapters had to gauge their response and decide what action or stance would be appropriate in response to the patient's agitated pacing, yelling, threatening to leave early, and so on.

I conclude now by quoting from an earlier paper by James McLaughlin (1981), in which he challenged the adult analyst:

> New knowledge of the complexity and content of transference has come to adult analyses from the fields of child and adolescent analysis and child development . . . and from studies of narcissistic and borderline patients. While they have broken no theoretical ground for countertransference, they have provided opportunity and challenge to the work-ego of the adult analyst to integrate both cognitive and experiential understandings of the range of separation–individuation experiences and the vicissitudes of narcissism in the patient himself. [p. 650]

The chapters contained in this book offer many such opportunities and challenges to all of us.

REFERENCES

Burlingham, D. (1935). Child analysis and the mother. *Psychoanalytic Quarterly* 4:69–92.
Cain, A. C., and Cain, B. S. (1964). On replacing a child. *Journal of the American Academy of Child Psychiatry* 3:443–456.
Edward, J., Ruskin, N., and Turrini, P. (1991). *Separation–Individuation Theory and Application*. New York: Gardner Press.
Frank, A. (1969). The unrememberable and the unforgettable: passive primal repression. *Psychoanalytic Study of the Child* 24:48–77. New York: International Universities Press.
Freud, S. (1916). Some character-types met with in psychoanalytic work. *Standard Edition* 14:311–336.
——— (1923). The ego and the id. *Standard Edition* 19:3–68.

—— (1924). The dissolution of the oedipus complex. *Standard Edition* 19:173–182.
—— (1925). Some psychical consequences of the anatomical differences between the sexes. *Standard Edition* 19:243–260.
Greenacre, P. (1971). Discussion of Eleanor Galenson's paper "A consideration of the nature of thought in childhood play." In *Separation–Individuation—Essays in Honor of Margaret S. Mahler*, ed. J. McDevitt and C. F. Settlage, pp. 60–69. New York: International Universities Press.
Greenson, R. (1968). Disidentifying from mother. *International Journal of Psycho-Analysis* 49:370–383.
Hoffer, W. (1952). The mutual influences in the development of the ego and the id. *Psychoanalytic Study of the Child* 7:31–42. New York: International Universities Press.
Jacobson, E. (1959). The "exception": an elaboration of Freud's character study. *Psychoanalytic Study of the Child* 14:135–142. New York: International Universities Press.
—— (1964). *The Self and Object World.* New York: International Universities Press.
Kay, P. (1978). Gifts, gratification, and frustration in child analysis. In *Child Analysis and Therapy*, ed. J. Glenn, pp. 309–354. New York: Jason Aronson.
Kramer, S. (1987). A contribution to the concept of "the exception" as a developmental phenomenon. *Child Abuse and Neglect* 11:367–370.
Kramer, S., and Akhtar, S. (1988). The developmental context of internalized preoedipal object relations: clinical applications of Mahler's theory of symbiosis and separation–individuation. *Psychoanalytic Quarterly* 57:547–576.
Kramer, S., and Byerly, L. (1978). Technique of psychoanalysis of the latency child. In *Child Analysis and Therapy*, ed. J. Glenn, pp. 205–233. New York: Jason Aronson.
Kris, E. (1956). The personal myth: a problem in psychoanalytic technique. *Journal of the American Psychoanalytic Association* 4:653–681.
Lebovici, S. (1973). *The current status of the infantile neurosis.* Paper presented at a panel for the Association for Child Psychoanalysis, Paris, July.
Loewald, H. (1974). Current status of the concept of infantile neurosis. *Psychoanalytic Study of the Child* 29:183–188. New York: International Universities Press.
Mahler, M. S. (1945). Child analysis. In *Modern Trend in Child Psychiatry*, ed. N. D. C. Lewis and B. Pacella, pp. 256–283. New York: International Universities Press.
—— (1974). Symbiosis and individuation: the psychological birth of the human infant. In *The Selected Papers of Margaret S. Mahler*, vol. 2, pp. 149–168. New York: Jason Aronson.
—— (1975). On the current status of the infantile neurosis. In *Selected Papers of Margaret S. Mahler*, vol. 2, pp. 189–192. New York: Jason Aronson.
Mahler, M. S., and McDevitt, J. (1980). The separation–individuation process and identity formation. In *The Course of Life, Infancy and Early Childhood*, vol. 1, ed. S. I. Greenspan and G. H. Pollock, pp. 395–406. Washington, DC: National Institute of Mental Health.
—— (1982). The emergence of the sense of self with particular emphasis on the body cells. *Journal of the American Psychoanalytic Association* 30:827–848.

Mahler, M. S., Pine, F., and Bergman, A. (1975). *The Psychological Birth of the Human Infant.* New York: Basic Books.

McLaughlin, J. (1981). Transference, psychic reality, and countertransference. *Psychoanalytic Quarterly* 50:639-664.

Parens, H. (1987). *Aggression in Our Children: Coping with It Constructively.* Northvale, NJ: Jason Aronson.

Poznanski, E. O. (1972). The replacement child: a saga of unresolved parental grief. *Behavioral Pediatrics* 81:1190-1193.

Riess, A. (1978). The mother's eye, for better or for worse. *Psychoanalytic Study of the Child* 33:381-409. New Haven: Yale University Press.

Ritvo, S. (1974). The current status of the infantile neurosis. *Psychoanalytic Study of the Child* 29:159-181. New York: International Universities Press.

Rosen, V. (1964). Some effects of artistic talents on character style. *Psychoanalytic Quarterly* 33:1-24.

Settlage, C. F. (1977). The psychoanalytic understanding of narcissistic and borderline personality disorders: advances in developmental theory. *Journal of the American Psychoanalytic Association* 25:805-833.

Stone, L. (1954). The widening scope of indications for psychoanalysis. *Journal of the American Psychoanalytic Association* 2:567-594.

Tolpin, M. (1980). Discussion of "psychoanalytic developmental theories of the self: an integration" by M. Shane and E. Shane. In *Advances in Self Psychology,* ed. A. Goldberg, pp. 47-68. New York: International Universities Press.

Weil, A. (1970). The basic core. *Psychoanalytic Study of the Child* 25:442-460. New York: International Universities Press.

2

TETHERS, ORBITS, AND INVISIBLE FENCES: CLINICAL, DEVELOPMENTAL, SOCIOCULTURAL, AND TECHNICAL ASPECTS OF OPTIMAL DISTANCE

Salman Akhtar, M.D.

"Anatomy is destiny" (Freud 1924, p. 178) and "the ego is first and foremost a bodily ego" (Freud 1923, p. 26) are two statements that epitomize Freud's lifelong stance toward humanity's corporeal existence. This stance was characterized by a deep and sustained regard for the somatic underpinnings of the intrapsychic, the interpersonal, and the cultural. Indeed psychoanalysis, the most profound method to study the human mind, was born in the course of Freud's investigating the puzzling somatic phenomenon of hysteria.

From then on, evidence of this intricate psychosomatic partnership in all other emotional disorders became undeniable. We became aware that the catatonics with their volitional disturbances, the paranoics with their somatic delusions, the hypochondriacs with their tenacious self-absorption, and the perverts and the addicts with their pleasurable corruption of the body's purposes are all calling our attention to this matter. We began noticing the milder signals from those not so obviously disturbed. Such clues from the day-to-day life include William

Shakespeare's "lean and hungry look," "bungled actions" (Freud 1905), postural oddities (F. Deutsch 1952), "neurotic bathing habits" (Fenichel 1945, p. 70), the peculiar "temperature and boundary sensitivity" of some individuals (Bach 1985, p. 21), those recurrent moments of unexplained nausea (Rossner 1983) and that "furtive pain around the mouth" (Wheelis 1966, p. 148) discernible in the prosperous crowd at a wine tasting or a private art exhibit. It is from these subtle reminders of psychosomatic unity that I have selected my topic: optimal distance.

In this chapter, I describe clinical manifestations of disturbed optimal distance, discuss the development of optimal distance and its pathology, and briefly comment upon the sociocultural vicissitudes of these phenomena. In addition, I provide some clinical material to highlight certain fantasies related to anxieties regarding distance and discuss the technical implications of the concept of distance. However, it seems best to begin by defining our terms.

DEFINITIONS

Distance: an interval or space between two points (Webster's New Universal Unabridged Dictionary, 2d ed.)

The terms "distance" and "optimal distance" do not appear in the index to the Standard Edition of Freud's works,[1] nor are

---

1. Freud used the word "distance" 92 times in his writings (Guttman, Jones, and Parish 1980). He spoke of tracing a train of thought for some "distance through consciousness" (1895, p. 300), the "distance between the object and the ego" (1915a, p. 137), something "at a distance from consciousness" (1915b, p. 203), the "distance between this ego ideal and the real ego" (1921, p. 110), and of an individual's putting "distance between himself and what is threatening him" (1926, p. 146) etc. Though these usages do occur in topographic, dynamic, structural, and adaptive contexts, the word "distance" is used colloquially and not as a scientific term itself.

they listed in the index to Fenichel's (1945) encyclopedic compilation of early psychoanalytic literature. Psychiatric (American Psychiatric Association 1975, Hinsie and Campbell 1975) and psychoanalytic (Laplanche and Pontalis 1973, Moore and Fine 1968, 1990, Rycroft 1972) glossaries also do not include these terms. This leaves one no option but to extrapolate the standard-use definitions of them (see above) to psychoanalytic theory. This, however, is no easy matter. For instance, the question immediately arises: Where is there an interval or space? Between two psychic structures? Between drives and defenses? Between self and object? Between self representation and object representation? Between two self representations? Between two object representations? Between the analyst and the analysand? And so on. Soon, the concept of distance begins to appear far from simple, and surely one cannot define "optimal distance" unless one decides what is meant by "distance."

In search of clarity one turns to earlier literature but finds that only two authors offer explicit definitions of the concept involved: Maurice Bouvet and Margaret Mahler. Bouvet (1958), in a pioneering paper entitled "Technical Variation and the Concept of Distance," defined "distance" as

> the gap [that] separates the way in which a subject expresses his instinctual drives from how he would express them if the process of "handling" or "managing" (in French: *amenagement*) these expressions did not intervene. [p. 211]

Bouvet goes on to explain that in his thinking this "managing"

> represents one aspect of the ego defenses, and this term seems to me useful since it draws attention to the *exterior aspect* of the ego's activity while "defense" characterizes more particularly its *internal aspect*. [p. 211, emphasis added]

A peculiar tension seems to exist in this definition. On the one hand, by regarding the gap between two manners of drive discharge as its cardinal characteristic, Bouvet posits an intrapsychic definition of the term "distance." On the other hand, by focusing on "managing" or the "exterior" aspect rather than on "defense" or the "internal" aspect of the ego's activity, Bouvet leans toward an interpersonal definition of "distance." This is more apparent in the following passage from the same paper.

> The distance [that] a patient will take from his analyst varies constantly during the analysis, but in general it tends to diminish as the analysis progresses, until it disappears. It is this point which I call the *rapprocher* (which signifies in French drawing close, but progressively). Once attained, this partial *rapprocher* can be jeopardized by other conflicts, but appears to be more easily reestablished, and to lead finally to a more general *rapprocher*. [pp. 211-212, author's emphasis]

Such two-sidedness of definition is also evident in the writings of Margaret Mahler. Interestingly, she begins her view of "distance" as being within the largely interpersonal mother-child matrix but ends up with an internalized capacity for establishing optimal distance, in other words, with an ego-attribute. "Optimal distance" for her is

> a position *between mother and child* that best allows the infant to develop those faculties which he needs in order to grow, that is, to individuate. [Mahler et al. 1975, p. 291, emphasis added]

This definition is an obviously interpersonal one. In other writings, however, Mahler (1971, 1975) takes a more intrapsychic perspective referring to the distance "between the self and the object world" (1975, p. 193). That she means *internalized* objects here is confirmed by the very next sentence, which refers to the

> oscillation between longing to merge with the good object representation, with the erstwhile (in one's fantasy at least) blissful

union with the symbiotic mother and the defense against reengulfment by her (which causes loss of autonomous self-identity). [1975, p. 193]

To my mind, both Bouvet and Mahler imply that "distance" is a Janus-faced concept with both intrapsychic and interpersonal referents.[2] One way out of this paradox is to define the concept only in one particular context at a time. In the developmental and therapeutic contexts the concept appears best defined in interpersonal terms, while in terms of individual psychodynamics it seems best defined intrapsychically. Another way is to follow Sandler's (1987) lead in defining projection not as the attribution of an unacceptable impulse to an outside agency but as its shifting from a self representation to an object representation. Accordingly, one could define distance as the space not between the self and the object but between the self representation and the object representation. Both these solutions resolve some conceptual difficulties and add others. A third solution is to not simplify things, to accept the paradox, and to regard the dialectical tension between two perspectives as being inherent to the phenomena involved. This is my preference, and a review of the factors contributing to the development of optimal distance tends to support my view.

DEVELOPMENTAL PERSPECTIVE

Despite the children's apparent obliviousness to their mother during the early practicing period, most of them seemed to go through a brief period of increased separation anxiety. The fact that they were able to move away independently, yet remain

---

2. This perhaps accounts for its lack of acceptance in psychoanalytic parlance. Moreover, to regard a distance as optimal involves a quantitative decision. This invokes the much disputed economic principle of metapsychology and renders the concept theoretically even more cumbersome.

connected with their mother—not physically, but by way of their seeing and hearing her—made the successful use of these distance modalities extra-ordinarily important. [Mahler 1974, pp. 157-158]

In 1959, Balint proposed two fundamental attitudes about distance from objects. These he termed the "ocnophilic" (hesitant, clinging) and the "philobatic" (thrill-loving) attitudes. Balint described the ocnophilic world as consisting of objects separated by horrid empty spaces and the philobatic world of friendly expanses dotted with unpredictable objects. The ocnophil lives from object to object, cutting short his travels through empty spaces. The philobat lives in friendly expanses, avoiding contact with potentially dangerous objects. The ocnophil feels safe as long as he is in touch with his objects, while the philobat lives in the illusion that he needs no objects. The ocnophil must please others. The philobat has no such need since he feels able to conquer the world without relying on potentially untrustworthy objects. The ocnophil likes to stay home; the philobat loves to travel. The two tendencies, however, never exist in isolation and their admixture is the rule.

In tracing their infantile origins, Balint at first regarded the ocnophilic tendency to be the earlier and the more primitive one. He felt that the philobatic attitude involves more skills and implies a greater acceptance of one's separate existence. However, a deeper look suggested the opposite to him. The ocnophil, in having to cling to others, betrays awareness of the gap between him and his objects, while the philobat seems to be living in a structureless, primitive state where there are few unimportant, unpredictable objects, a world that consists only of kindly substances, constituting the friendly expanses. His world is "a kind of loving mother holding her child safely in her arms" (pp. 84-85).

While I follow Balint's second formulation, that is, that the philobatic attitude is earlier than the ocnophilic one, I find his first formulation (which suggests the reverse) theoretically more sound. His own statement supports this. Balint finds that whereas "the ocnophilic world is structured by physical proximity and touch, the philobatic world is structured by safe distance and sight" Balint (p. 34). In other words, the ocnophilic attitude implies lesser separation from primary objects, especially the mother, than does the philobatic attitude. This makes the former seem the developmentally earlier one. Such thinking is supported by the observation that the shift from tactile to visual modality for contact with mother originates in experiences of separation.[3] Spitz (1965) observes that

> when the infant loses the nipple and recovers it, contact with the need-gratifying percept is lost and recovered, and lost and recovered, again and again. During the interval between loss and recovery of *contact* the other element of the total perceptual unit, *distance perception* of the face, remains unchanged. In the course of these repetitive experiences visual perception comes to be relied upon, for it is not lost; it proves to be the more constant and therefore the more rewarding of the two. [p. 65, author's emphasis]

Thus philobatism, which relies heavily on vision, seems an attitude more accepting of separation than ocnophilia, which demands physical contact. The close correspondence between Balint's ocnophilic and philobatic attitudes and Mahler's symbiotic and practicing phases (Mahler 1965, 1971, 1972, Mahler et al. 1975) respectively upholds this view. Balint's acknowledgment of the ubiquitous coexistence of these attitudes echoes in Mahler's recognition of "man's eternal struggle against both fusion and isolation" (Mahler 1972, p. 130). Balint's describing the occasionally painful tension between ocnophilic and philobatic attitudes within an individual parallels Mahler's (1971,

---

3. Greenacre (1953) may have been first to note this connection in describing the "uncanny reaching out with the eyes" (p. 90) of children not sufficiently held and cuddled by their mothers.

Tethers, Orbits, and Invisible Fences

1974) conceptualization of "rapprochement crisis" and its reverberations in certain character constellations.

Let me take a few steps back, however, and point out that Mahler posits that at the beginning of life and for the first four to five months (the symbiotic stage) the mother and infant constitute a dual unity. There is no outside world for the infant. Gradually, however, there develops "the space between mother and child" (Bergman 1980, p. 201).[4] This is partly created by the mother's comings and goings and partly by a decrease in the baby's bodily dependence on the mother, permitting him to look "beyond the symbiotic orbit" (Mahler 1974, p. 155). During this, the differentiation subphase of separation-individuation (from 4 to 10 months), the infant attempts to break away, in a bodily sense, from the hitherto passive lap-babyhood.

> All infants like to venture and stay just a bit of a distance away from the enveloping arms of the mother; and, as soon as they are motorically able to, they like to slide down from the mother's lap. But they tend to remain or crawl back, as near as possible, to play at the mother's feet. [Mahler 1974, p. 155]

It is during the practicing subphase (from 10 to 18 months), however, that the child shows greater ability to move away from the mother, at first by crawling and later by upright locomotion. The child makes pleasurable forays in the external world, is enamored by his burgeoning ego capacities, and seems oblivious to the mother's presence.[5] Yet, revealing his continued need for a "home base," he periodically returns to the mother.

---

4. Winnicott (1971) is also interested in this space. However, his focus is not upon the child's ambivalent efforts to minimize it but upon its persistence and varying psychic uses throughout life.

5. Gender differences exist in the extent of this distance. Little girls have a "lesser degree of motor-mindedness" (Mahler et al. 1975, p. 214) and do not venture as far from their mothers as do boys of similar age. Moreover, the distance that mothers comfortably permit their little children to move away is almost always shorter than that allowed by fathers (Pruett 1990).

Gradually, the cognitive strides made by the child make him all too aware of his smallness, of his separateness, and of the fact that he cannot coerce his mother to gratify his every need. His previously enjoyed fantasies of shared omnipotence collapse. The child is now in the rapprochement subphase (from 18 to 24 months). Ambivalence and ambitendency prevail. Much intrapsychic conflict is produced by the coexisting progressive desires for self-assertion, separation, and autonomy on the one hand and regressive wishes for closeness, even symbiotic merger with his mother, on the other hand. There develops a tendency toward mood swings. No distance from mother appears satisfactory. Closeness soothes narcissistic wounds but stirs up the dread of fusion. Being apart enhances pride but leaves one lonely. Contradictory demands are made upon the mother. If the mother remains emotionally available despite such oscillations on the part of the child, then there occurs a gradual mending of contradictory object (the mother of symbiosis and the mother of separation) and self (the "lap baby" of symbiosis and the "conqueror" of practicing) representations. Capacity for object and self constancy develops, along with a capacity for maintaining optimal distance. However, if the mother is not optimally available during the rapprochement subphase, these developmental achievements do not result. The contradictory self and object representations remain split, infantile omnipotence is not renunciated, and capacity for optimal distance fails to develop. This leads to a lifelong tendency toward oscillation between passionate intimacy and hateful withdrawal from objects.

In light of this, optimal distance is best viewed as a psychic position that permits intimacy without loss of autonomy and separateness without painful aloneness. This definition, though not clearly spelled out by Mahler in the context of adult character organization, is, I believe, the essence of her position on this matter. Having thus enriched the definition of optimal distance from a developmental perspective, we are now prepared to discuss its disturbances.

PSYCHOPATHOLOGY OF OPTIMAL DISTANCE

A number of porcupines huddled together for warmth on a cold day in winter; but, as they began to prick one another with their quills, they were obliged to disperse. However the cold drove them together again, when just the same thing happened. At last, after many turns of huddling and dispersing, they discovered that they would be best off by remaining at a little distance from one another. [Schopenhauer 1981, p. 226]

Many psychopathological syndromes are characterized by behaviors suggestive of difficulty in maintaining optimal distance. A prominent example is agoraphobia, which typically involves a "fearful aversion to leaving familiar surroundings" (Roth 1959) unless accompanied by a reassuring companion. While this is often the end product of the repressed prostitution fantasy identified by Freud (1892-1899: 1897 extract, p. 253), other dynamic factors also play a role in its causation. In an early paper on "locomotor anxiety," Abraham (1913) noted that neurotic inhibitions of motility emanate not only from defenses against constitutionally strong pleasure in movement and unconscious sexual concerns but also from difficulty in separating from love objects. Some years later, Helene Deutsch (1929) declared the involvement of a partner to be the crucial determinant of the agoraphobic's malady. However, she felt that hostile and controlling fantasies were frequently hidden underneath the consciously experienced need for libidinal attachment. Following this, Mittleman (1957) observed the confinement of the agoraphobic to a "limited circumference" (p. 289), and Weiss (1964) noted that such patients grow more anxious the farther they go from their homes. This led him to define "agoraphobia" as "an anxiety reaction to abandoning a fixed point of support." More recently, Kohut (1980) concluded that the agoraphobic's consciously felt need for a reassuring companion is the key to what lies in his psychic depths, namely, the continued search for a maternal self-object. Clearly, all these authors regard agoraphobia as a malady of distance. How far can one go away from one's objects without endangering the integrity of one's self?

Contributing to claustrophobia is the opposite question. How close can one get to another person without risking one's autonomy? An alternate activation of these concerns is evident in certain chronic marital difficulties. Like Schopenhauer's porcupines (Barnes 1981), the two partners fluctuate between intimacy and distance, trust and mistrust, betrayal and confession, and separation and reunion. They cannot live peacefully together, nor can they do without each other. They lack the capacity to establish complementarity of roles and are unable to follow Gibran's (1923) counsel for marital partners to

> stand together yet not too near together:
>
> For the pillars of the temple stand apart, and the oak tree and the cypress grow not in each other's shadow. [p. 16]

Although the proximity afforded by marriage does play a triggering role, such hopeless failure in negotiating an optimal distance almost invariably betrays separate character pathology in the two partners. Actually, severe personality disorders constitute the cardinal example of psychopathology involving optimal distance. Included here are narcissistic, borderline, schizoid, paranoid, hypomanic (Akhtar 1988), infantile or histrionic, as-if (H. Deutsch 1942), and antisocial personality disorders. For such individuals, involvement with others stirs up a characteristic "need–fear dilemma" (Burnham, et al. 1969): to be intimate is to risk engulfment, and to be apart is to court aloneness. This leads to a variety of compromises. The borderline continues to go back and forth (Akhtar 1990, Gunderson 1985, Melges and Swartz 1989). The narcissist can sustain allegiances longer and therefore shows such oscillations less often (Adler 1981, Akhtar 1989, Kernberg 1970). The paranoid individual bristles at any change in distance initiated by others (Akhtar 1990a), preferring

the "reliability" of his fear of being betrayed (Blum 1981). The schizoid individual opts for withdrawal on the surface while maintaining an intense imaginative tie to his objects (Akhtar 1987, Fairbairn 1952, Guntrip 1969). Antisocial and hypomanic individuals, though internally uncommitted, develop rapid intimacy with others. This tendency to be highly attuned to others, even magically identifying with them, is most evident in the "as-if" personalities (Deutsch 1942) and underlies the fraudulent tendency in these and other individuals (Gediman 1985).

I would like to emphasize, however, that agoraphobia, marital difficulties, and severe personality disorders display the most overt difficulties of optimal distance. More subtle anxieties in this realm become discernible only during psychoanalytic work. Here the ebb and flow of the associative material and evolving transferences frequently reveal anxieties pertaining to distance and closeness, as well as fantasies defending against these anxieties.

THE TETHER FANTASY AND ITS VARIANTS

The child had a wooden reel with a piece of string tied round it. It never occurred to him to pull it along the floor behind him, for instance, and play at its being a carriage. What he did was to hold the reel by the string and very skillfully throw it over the edge of his curtained cot, so that it disappeared into it, at the same time uttering his expressive "o-o-o-o." He then pulled the reel out of the cot again by the string and hailed its reappearance with a joyful "da" ["there"]. This, then, was the complete game—disappearance and return.... It was related to the child's great cultural achievement—the instinctual renunciation (that is, the renunciation of instinctual satisfaction) which he had made in allowing his mother to go away without protesting. He compensated himself for this, as it were, by himself staging the disappearance and return to the objects within his reach. [Freud 1920, p. 15]

One such fantasy is that of a tether, that is, a rope or chain that keeps one within certain bounds. While only one analysand referred to it literally as such, three other patients reported essentially similar fantasies. In all four instances, the fantasy defended against anxiety regarding distance and seemed to have links with the rapprochement subphase of separation–individuation (Mahler 1971, 1975, Mahler et al. 1975). However, there are a few caveats. First, these fantasies should not be taken as representing the actual ideational events of the latter half of the second year of life. While "the unrememberable and the unforgettable" (Frank 1969) affects and wordless thoughts of that period do form the building blocks of these fantasies, their specific content requires greater cognitive maturity and appears derived from later childhood. Second, the manner in which these fantasies are communicated (by the patient) and deciphered (by the analyst) makes certainty about them difficult. Pertaining largely to the preverbal period, these are hardly ever well put into words. Patients resort to allusions and metaphors, while the analysts find themselves relying to a greater than usual extent upon their own affective experience (Akhtar 1991, Burland 1975). The ground is murky and clarity is in short supply. Third, while the tether fantasy and its variants seem related to rapprochement-subphase issues, in accordance with the principle of multiple function (Waelder 1930), they also contain drive-defense-type conflicts from various psychosexual levels, including the phallic-oedipal phase. The issue of distance is also paramount during the oedipal phase,[6] and these fantasies often

---

6. The establishment of the incest barrier is an apt illustration of the relevance of distance during the oedipal phase. However, "the task of mastering the oedipal complex is not simply to renounce primary oedipal objects, but to do so in a way that simultaneously permits individual autonomy together with maintenance of valued traditional continuity" (Poland 1977, p. 410). Moreover, the prohibition of sexual transgression resulting from this phase need not eliminate aim-inhibited, subtle affirma-

have parallel meanings derived from that context. Finally, the fantasies' potentially idiosyncratic relevance for a given patient should also be considered. With these caveats, let me proceed to the tether fantasy.

Case 1

This was first brought to my attention by Mr. B., a successful, twice-divorced businessman in his mid-forties. Mr. B. had sought analysis because he was again considering marriage and was afraid about its outcome. Initial interviews suggested that Mr. B. often fell in love with needy women who had a "faint breath of scandal" (Freud 1910, p. 166) about them and lost interest in them after his rescue of them. This oedipal dynamic seemed to have a solid footing on his account of a reasonably peaceful early childhood; an excessively conscientious latency; and a family constellation of a rebellious older brother, an admired but distant father, and a very involved, somewhat anxious mother. However, there were also hints of anxiety in Mr. B. about separation and fusion. On the one hand, he had broken off his marriages because of feeling "suffocated"; on the other hand, he was not able to give up anything.

Mr. B. began analysis with the fervor of the dedicated student he always had been. He worked hard at it, talked incessantly, and was quick to identify with my analyzing style. His concerns about separation showed in many ways. He expressed a fear of never being able to leave analysis, do nothing but analysis, become an "analytic monk." At the end of each session, he would get up, look at me—as if taking me in for safekeeping—and announce our next appointment with a subtle questioning tone at the end. (This often extracted a nod from me but was not brought into analysis for quite a while.)

---

tion of attractiveness between parents and children. Indeed, there might exist an "oedipally optimal" optimal distance, that is, a distance between two generations that is neither incestuously intrusive nor oblivious of each other's attractiveness.

The tether fantasy appeared in the third month of his analysis. One day he announced that he was going away to a sales meeting on the West Coast, adding in the same breath that his attendance there was not mandatory. I pointed out his ambivalence and commented on the anxiety he seemed to be experiencing with his wish to be temporarily away and thus be separated from me. He agreed and said that he wanted somehow to be at both places simultaneously. Further associations during this and later sessions revealed that he frequently had difficulty leaving places, people, even ideas and options. He was never fully at one place and often carried something of where he had formerly been with him. As the day of his departure drew closer, Mr. B. became more anxious. He started fearing being so far away from my office and from me. He had disturbing thoughts about feeling hungry late at night while staying in a hotel on the West Coast, not being able to find any food in the lobby, going hungry, and dying of starvation.

It was around this time that Mr. B. first reported the fantasy of a tether, a long rope by which he was tied to my office while being on the West Coast. With this he could be there safely and feel much less anxiety. As he was talking about this, he visualized a little boy learning to walk. As is often typical of visual images during analytic sessions (Warren 1961), this picture was at first affectless and experienced as having little or no connection with the patient's own self. Gradually, however, Mr. B. was able to acknowledge more directly both the anxiety and the pleasure in his wish to walk away from me. The imagined tether clearly served a defensive purpose insofar as it minimized the anxiety of separation while permitting him autonomous functioning.

During later periods of Mr. B.'s analysis, the fantasied tether reappeared off and on around separations. While in the beginning only its reassuring aspects were evident, ambivalence gradually became attached to it. At times, it felt like an enslaving chain from which he wanted escape. Were he not tied to me, he could go have more fun, have sex with more women! Such associations gradually propelled Mr. B.'s analysis to more familiar oedipal themes. The tether disappeared from his associations, became irrelevant. During termination Mr. B. did recall the tether, however. This was associated with jocular disbelief, which at times seemed to hide a wistful longing for continued attachment to me. At other times, his humor displayed pleasure in his increased psychic freedom both within himself and in relation to me.

Less graphic but similar themes were reported by three other patients:

Case 2

Ms. D. felt that an "invisible fence" precluded too much movement on her part. It prevented her from taking up a better job at a location about 4 miles farther from her current place of employment and from my office. Significant assertiveness of any sort, especially vis-à-vis her domineering and controlling mother (and later toward me), led her to feel a jolting "electric shock." She said that she felt like a dog in a yard with an invisible electric fence. "I can only go this far, but if I try to hit the street I get the shock." The idea of "hitting the street" led her to think of leaving home, as well as to "street walking" and loss of control of sexual impulses. Further analysis revealed a childhood of intense engulfment by an exhibitionistic, hypochondriacal, and controlling mother, and marked inattention from a self-engrossed, heavily drinking father.

Case 3

Mr. E., a young college student who, as far back as he could remember, had felt "completely forgotten" by his mother, reported many social and motoric inhibitions. One among these was his anxiety about jogging. While he enjoyed jogging, he constantly worried that he would end up too far away from his home, get hopelessly lost, and be unable to find his way back. As a result, he jogged only around the block, never permitting himself to go "too far away" from his apartment building.

Case 4

Ms. F. felt a similar inhibition in mental activities. A politically conscious attorney who at the age of 18 months had been separated from her mother for about six to eight weeks, Ms. F. had never felt close to her mother. While growing up she felt her mother to be an "all duty and no love" type of person who pushed Ms. F. toward premature independence. As a child she feared acquiring skills, since it led to greater autonomy and loss of attention from her mother. Further exploration revealed that she found reading fiction especially difficult, since rapt absorption took her "away" from her surroundings. In the midst of reading a "fat novel" (an unmistakable reference to the oral-visual incorporative axis), for instance, she would suddenly become aware of her absorption and start to worry lest she get "lost" in reading at the expense of other chores. It was as if she had stretched her mental tether to the limit and had to return to the secure base of reality for refueling.

Common to these patients was their concern about distance from an anchoring person or environment. They felt confined to an orbit. Upon reaching the outer limit of this orbit, they felt anxious and retreated to a comfortable distance within it. They felt reassured by a central point of reference and feared getting lost if they broke the tether by going "too far." At times, however, they experienced a hypomaniclike excitement at the thought of this eventuality. Mr. E., for instance, imagined that if he allowed himself to jog freely, he might go on for 100 or 200 miles, perhaps even farther. Ms. F. felt that if she allowed herself to read with concentration, she might keep reading, miss her work, and disregard her analytic appointments. In such moments, real or imagined, these patients were flooded with elation and grandiosity, covered over during the analytic sessions by slightly apologetic giggling and shyness.

Their concerns were strongly reminiscent of those experienced by children in the practicing and rapprochement subphase of separation–individuation. The main issue here is that of distance versus safety. Although distancing from mother begins in the differentiation subphase, it is not until the practicing and rapprochement subphases that the "symbiotic orbit" (Mahler et al. 1975, p. 293) actually begins to be mapped out and the strength of the "invisible bond" (p. 25) between mother and child is truly tested. Mr. B., in feeling reassured that a tether connected him to me while he traveled, was like a toddler in the practicing subphase. During this time, despite pleasurable forays in the external world, the "mother continues to be needed as a stable point, a 'home base' to fulfill the need for refueling" (Mahler et al. 1975, p. 69). Mr. E.'s and Ms. F.'s hypomanic excitement while at the furthest extremes of their tethers also resembled practicing-phase children's elation upon freely exercising their ego apparatuses and escaping from fusion with the mother. These patients also showed the characteristic ambitendency of rapprochement-subphase children. They wanted to assert themselves and experiment with a wider segment of the world but feared losing touch with the "home base." At the same time, they feared moving too close to the center of their orbit (note Mr. B.'s fear of becoming an "analytic monk"). Fearing both progression and regression, they existed in a "satellite state" (Volkan and Corney 1968), that is, as captive bodies orbiting within the gravitational field of an intense, though ambivalent, dependency. Their distancing attempts (e.g., travels, jogging, assertiveness) reassured them against the dread of fusion while their imaginary tethers provided them "distance contact" (Mahler et al. 1975, p. 67) with the analyst, who remained available despite their comings and goings. It gave them time to work out both their separation anxiety and their dread of merger and to negotiate an optimal distance from early maternal object representations and their transferential recreations during analysis.

To the best of my knowledge, the tether fantasy described here is not mentioned in the psychoanalytic literature. However, there do exist three accounts of children with similar undertones. Freud's (1920) description of his grandson's playing with a wooden reel, which serves as the epigraph of this section of the chapter, seems to refer to an enactment of the tether fantasy. Following Freud, Winnicott (1960a) reported the case of a 7-year-old boy who was preoccupied with strings and was constantly tying up various household objects to each other. In view of the child's many traumatic separations from his mother beginning around the age of 3, Winnicott felt that the boy was "attempting to deny separation by his use of string, as one would deny separation from a friend by using the telephone" (p. 154). More recently Fischer (1991) noted the preoccupation with a "transatlantic cable" in an 8-year-old boy facing separation from his analyst and worrying about the latter's whereabouts during their summer break.

Besides being particularly apt as a metaphor in this regard, the fantasy of a tether may also have contributions from childhood realities.[7] The joining functions of strings and ropes are routinely witnessed by children. They may see pets on leashes and farm animals on tethers. They play with yo-yos and other string-manipulated toys. Toddlers in stores are sometimes restrained by "leashes" held by harried parents. Kindergarten children on school-sponsored field trips often hold on to a rope whose end is held by their teacher. Thus there are ample opportunities for ropes, leashes, tethers, and strings to be incorporated in inner concerns about maintaining contact with someone while being physically apart.[8]

---

7. Issues from other levels may also contribute to the tether fantasy. Two such examples are, at the deepest, "prehistoric" level, the somatic schemata involving the umbilical cord and, at the highest, most elaborate level, the imagoes of maternal phallus.

8. Ropes, strings, and chains have been used throughout history as symbols for binding and connection (Cirlot 1971). The sacred thread *(Janaiyu)* worn across their chests by all high-caste Hindus is the external

Colloquial wisdom seems aware of the kinship between metaphor and reality in this regard. This is evident in such expressions as "He's tied to his mother's apron strings," "He has her on a leash," "He hasn't been able to cut the cord yet," and "She's at the end of her rope." Such linguistic clues bring us to other significant reverberations of distance and closeness in the sociocultural realm.

SOCIOCULTURAL VICISSITUDES

And when the shadow fades and is no more, the light that lingers becomes a shadow to another light.

And thus your freedom when it loses its fetters becomes itself the fetter of a greater freedom. [Gibran 1923, p. 49]

Conflicts regarding distance can also be discerned in three sociocultural realms: (1) childhood games and amusement park rides, (2) travel and vacations, and (3) migration and exile. A closer look at each of these realms reveals the common intrapsychic denominator of distance, although with varying magnitude and different results.

1. Childhood Games and Amusement Park Rides. Prominent among the multiple determinants of childhood games (Balint 1959, Erikson 1950, Freud 1920, Glenn 1991, Kleeman 1967, Phillips 1960, Waelder 1933, Winnicott 1971) is the attempt to master anxiety about separation and loss. Peekaboo, the universal childhood game initiated by the mother during the

---

symbol of things in existence. The Egyptian hieroglyphic of a vertical chain of three links with the bottom link left open holds dual symbolism. On the one hand, it signifies the evolution and involution of the heaven and earth, and on the other hand, the matrimony between man and woman. Perhaps all sashes, bows, braids, and stripes worn by soldiers and officials are, besides being obvious phallic symbols, emblems of cohesion.

differentiation subphase and resumed vigorously by the child during rapprochement (Kleeman 1967, Mahler 1971, 1972, Mahler et al. 1975), is mostly aimed at fostering tolerance of separation from the mother. The child's pleasure in it comes from his rediscovering the mother after a brief, tense moment of losing her. This theme of losing and regaining safety also underlies later, more formal games of latency, though clearly these also have prominent phallic-oedipal undercurrents (Glenn 1991). All these games involve leaving a zone of safety, courting danger more or less voluntarily, and returning to the secure zone (almost always called "home"). Attempts at mastering separation anxiety are clearly evident here. At the same time, these games permit the player, rather like the rapprochement-phase toddler, the vicarious enjoyment of both merger and separateness from the "home base," that is, mother.

A similar "mixture of fear, pleasure, and confident hope in face of an external danger is what constitutes the fundamental nature of all *thrills*" (Balint 1959, p. 23). This is nowhere more evident than at amusement parks. The rides offered there involve high speeds, exposed situations, tunnels, darkness, giddiness and vertigo, and unfamiliar angles. By exposing the thrill seeker to physical danger and then returning him unhurt, such rides serve as counterphobic reassurances against castration anxiety. However, by removing an individual from familiar and safe ground (home, mother) and then returning him to it, these rides also capitalize on libidinization of separation-related fears.

2. Travel and Vacations. Actual travel powerfully activates distance-related anxieties (Chmiel et al. 1979). Some people travel easily, while others are homebound (Balint 1959). Some enjoy traveling a shade too much, raising suspicions of counterphobic mechanisms at work. Still others are literally vagabonds and hoboes, hopelessly unable to stay put. All these individuals betray conflicts over distance from their love objects.

In the midst of such conflicted attitudes is the social institution of vacations. In a thoughtful exposition on the dynamic, economic, structural, and adoptive correlates of a "good" vacation, Grinstein (1955) somehow omits the issue of distance from home. This is important in two ways here. First, the distance to which one can go for a "vacation" unaccompanied by one's loved ones is much shorter (in time and space) than the one traveled in their company. Second, there seems to be an optimal distance from home needed to have a good time. We cannot have a relaxing vacation in a hotel five miles from home, nor can we go too far away (using the rationalization that such places lack adequate resources to sustain us). We need to go away yet remain within a certain boundary.[9]

3. Migration and Exile. The issue of distance is of extreme relevance to the situation of the immigrant. Leaving one's country involves profound losses. Often one has to give up familiar foods, native music, even one's language ("mother tongue"). The new country offers strange-tasting foods, new songs, different political concerns, unfamiliar language, awkward attires, pale festivals, unknown heroes, unearned history, and visually unfamiliar landscapes. The immigrant finds himself at too much distance from the land of those constituting his multilayered internal objects, that is, his ancestors ("My lands are where my dead lie buried," proclaimed Crazy Horse; quoted in Dewall 1984, p. 26). He lacks the "refueling" privilege of college students who return to parental homes with an unspoken regularity (typically around occasions that offer sumptuous meals). Immigration experience seems to constitute a "third individuation," although deeper attention at an individual im-

---

9. Such extension of the boundary of one's home, as it were, is also discernible in certain religious concessions. For instance, the Hebrew laws of eruv are meant to facilitate locomotor freedom and enhance carrying privileges on Sabbath (Kaplan 1971). These laws involve the symbolic creation of new "home bases" along the way, thus extending the boundary of one's original dwelling. I am thankful to Jeanne Meisler, M.D., for bringing this to my attention.

migrant's dynamics may indeed reveal it to be simultaneously a continuation of the "second individuation of adolescence" (Blos 1967).

The "psychic pain" (Freud 1926, p. 169) caused by the distance between the immigrant's first and second homes leads to fluctuations between intense nostalgia for the lost land and anxious setting of roots in the new culture. Homesickness in this connection contains at its kernel a longing for the mother's breast (Sterba 1940). Fantasies of "someday" (Akhtar 1991) returning to one's earlier home (mother) sustain the immigrant through the mourning (Grinberg and Grinberg 1989, Pollock 1989) warranted by separation from it. A frequent stopgap measure is actual travel back to the country of origin for refueling purposes. Carrying back gifts to the relatives left behind, and bringing artifacts, childhood mementos, and old photographs upon return to the new home, the immigrant reminds one of a growing child crisscrossing the space between himself and his mother. The following observations of Bergman (1980), though made in connection with the young child, seem equally applicable to the immigrant.

> As... he is able to move away farther, his world begins to widen, there is more to see, more to hear, more to touch, and each time he returns to mother he brings with him some of the new experience. In other words, each time he returns he is ever so slightly changed. The mother is the center of his universe to whom he returns as the circles of his exploration widen. [p. 203]

The distance between two lands (two mothers, i.e., the "mother of symbiosis" and the "mother of separation") is also bridged by developing homoethnic ties in the new country, and by making use of the radio or cassette player to listen to one's own music. These serve as "transitional objects" (Winnicott 1953) and facilitate a progressive move in the mourning process consequent upon migration. Clearly, this mourning is not only for important love objects but also for "lost parts of the self" (Grinberg and Grinberg 1984, p. 13).

At the same time, migration provides an opportunity for psychic expansion, growth, and alteration. New channels of self-expression become available. There are new identification models, different superego prohibitions, different ideals. Ethnocentric clinging to fellow immigrants or a chameleonlike identity change are two problematic outcomes (Teja and Akhtar 1981) of the failure to negotiate the distance between the old and the emerging self representations. An optimal distance facilitates synthesis, leading to the emergence of a new hybrid identity. Such identity might lack deep anchoring in either historical and identification systems but may possess a greater than usual breadth of experience, knowledge, and, at times, wisdom.

The situation is, of course, much more complex with involuntary migration. Individuals who had to flee from the Nazis, from Latin America, from Haiti, from Cuba, and more recently from Cambodia, Laos, and Vietnam often cannot ever return to their lands of origins. This blocks access to refueling. The child within is orphaned and must reclaim inch by inch (with the aid of old photographs, music, books, relics, news, and above all new transferences, introspection, and creativity) the psychic territory lost. Such a mourning process may, however, last a lifetime and even then be incomplete.

All in all it seems that (1) childhood games and amusement park rides involve relatively "safer" journeys to and from love objects; (2) travel and vacations stretch the tether and map out the outer limits of the symbiotic orbit; there is a lot of fun to be had, but one has to return; and (3) migration involves a loss of "home base," a mourning over it, and a creation of a new home and a hybrid self; exile is a "malignant" form of migration where refueling is not possible, practicing is aborted, and mourning is incomplete. This digression into the sociocultural realm, however, must not take us away from the fact that the issue of distance is basically an intrapsychic one. It has ontogenetic roots, pathological presentations, and, above all, implications for the technique of psychoanalysis and intensive psychotherapy.

TECHNICAL IMPLICATIONS OF THE CONCEPT OF DISTANCE

Tact derives from separation experiences. Here the model is literally that of the mother's soothing touch. It extends, of course, beyond touch to all modalities available for the infant's experience of the mothering one in that early phase. In particular, we think of the quality of the analyst's warmth, not the excessive warmth of denied hostility, but the basic readiness of the analyst to be available to understand the patient. The tact of the analyst is a highly refined technical correlate of the physician's well-known art of "laying on of the hands." [Poland 1975, p. 157]

The concept of distance has many technical implications. These implications affect our work from its beginning until its end, perhaps even afterwards. For instance, during an initial consultation in which the recommendation of an analysis is going to be made, it is of utmost importance that the consultant avoid any premature closeness with the patient. Most concretely, this applies to not answering factually those questions of the patient that pertain to the analyst's personality around which transference would develop. Another early situation that warrants exploration instead of a quick reality decision is when a patient declares that he will be leaving town in two, three, or even four years. Such "realities" often involve anxiety about closeness. This needs to be gently brought up for discussion and not permitted to compromise the open-ended nature of commitment for psychoanalysis.

A more subtle issue during the initial consultation, however, involves making sure that a recommendation of analysis is not confused by the patient with a recommendation of analysis with the consultant (Klauber 1971). This confusion is the basis of much narcissistic injury to the patient when a referral to a colleague is made and may even cause difficulties in subsequent treatment. Confusion is more likely to occur during initial evaluations with "famous" analysts (with whom an idealizing patient brings himself too close too quickly) or with "charismatic" analysts (who for stylistic and characterological reasons may bring the patient too close to themselves too quickly). It is possible that an early supervisor of mine had such distance issues in mind when he suggested an alternate way of asking the same question. The patient, a man in his mid-twenties, was talking in his second or third consultation session with me about his ambivalent feelings toward recent Asian immigrants. After listening for a while, I asked him how he felt about being in any kind of treatment with me (an Asian immigrant). My supervisor remarked that rather than saying, "How might you feel being in treatment with me?" I could have said, "How might you feel being in treatment with someone you might recognize as an immigrant?" The latter question is less personal and therefore allows the patient greater freedom of expression. To have made no comment upon the patient's associations would have created too much distance (i.e., leaving him no choice but to drop the subject), but to comment as I did left the patient too little distance (forcing him to address its unacceptable transference significance). My supervisor's stance facilitated optimal distance.

Another early situation that brings up the issue of distance is when a patient gives up sitting and begins to lie down on the couch. The ensuing loss of visual contact increases the distance from the analyst. The analyst then has to be mindful of the effects of this upon the patient's feeling states and ego capacities, as well as of the defensive strategies mobilized by the patient to compensate for this increased distance. Talking rapidly and incessantly to seek contact with the analyst, curling up in a frightened ball to hold on to oneself, asking provocative questions and mumbling inaudibly to evoke activity from the analyst, and focusing on the details of the office as a derivative of the wish to maintain visual contact with the analyst, are all manifestations that betray anxiety over this increased distance and should be interpreted as such. Unusual manifestations of anxieties pertaining to this sudden increase in distance should also be kept in mind. Ms. D., for instance, began to lie on the couch so that a significant portion of her face was visible to me, and I found myself repeatedly looking at her. The interpretation of this situation appeared multidetermined and included her childhood overstimulation by parental nudity. However, this reversal of anxious scopophilia into teasing exhibitionism was also linked to her distress at losing visual contact with me.

Many questions arise here. Do patients who have sat up for long periods before using the couch react more or less intensely, similarly, or differently to lying down? Are there patients who should not be kept sitting up for long because the distance might become socially too close or, conversely, fixated in a more than optimal apartness from their deepest, inner lives? Should some patients be seen at first sitting up, even four or five sessions a week, for a long period of time so that they can establish a "reality base" (Volkan 1987, p. 85) about the analyst's personality necessary for them to avoid dangerous transference regressions? Finally, can the analyst undertake active measures, besides the usual empathic remarks and clarifications, to minimize the patient's distress on beginning to use the couch? Some analysts do report an early "noisy phase" (Boyer 1967, Volkan 1987, p. 87) when they grunt more than usual to assure their sicker patients of their continued involvement. What do we think of this? Or of Winnicott's remark at the end of the first session of Guntrip's analysis with him? Winnicott remained totally silent throughout the session and said at the end, "I've nothing particular to say yet, but if I don't say something, you may begin to feel I'm not here" (Guntrip 1975 p. 152).

The significance of the issue of distance is not restricted to the initial evaluation and the beginning phase. It appears again and again in the course of our work. Indeed, with some patients this happens so often that we might conclude that when the issue is not overtly present it is being adequately addressed. For instance, if we move a bit closer to the couch and lean forward to make a point, we may encroach painfully upon these patients. The optimal distance which was until that moment taken for granted is suddenly ruptured, and an "impingement" (Winnicott 1960b) results. This often detours the course of analytic work. Conversely, not acting on a patient's behalf at times painfully increases the distance. Here I am reminded of an analytic patient who, because of a coughing fit, was having much difficulty talking and asked me where she could get a glass of water. I helped her obtain a glass of water (we had just moved into a new office building and water fountains had not yet been turned on). I wondered about the effects of my doing this but felt that not doing so would have highlighted my abstinent stance too much, increased the distance between us, and rendered me realistically intrusive and transferentially unusable.

Similar considerations apply to the analyst's vacations and to accidental meetings between the analyst and the analysand outside the office. Both alter the distance between the two parties. Vacations tend to put the analyst "too far" and accidental encounters "too close." Both the analyst and the patient are put to some test under such circumstances. While clearly the optimal distance in such circumstances varies with various analyst–patient dyads, and perhaps also from early to middle to final phases of analysis, it remains the analyst's responsibility to safeguard this optimal distance.

Even outside such unusual situations, the concept of optimal distance is of utmost importance to analytic technique. For instance, a proper mixture of experiencing and observing on the part of our patients facilitates the analytic work. In other words, a patient's ego takes an equidistant position from affects and intellect, known and unknown, past and present, and transference distortion and therapeutic alliance. Similarly, for maintaining his neutrality, the analyst is advised to be "equidistant"

(A. Freud 1936, p. 38) from the patient's id, reality, and superego concerns. The concept of distance is equally applicable to interpretation, especially the "mutative interpretations" (Strachey 1934) that lead to an enlightenment through experience

> or a coming together which establishes the identity between a present emotional experience and its prototype in the past, and requires the coming together of the unconscious of the analyst and patient, thus making possible a revelation which affirms the *rapprocher*. . . . The tone and the form in which it is expressed are dictated by the necessity of not breaking this *rapprocher*, still in a potential state, but on the contrary of reinforcing it. Of equal importance, as already noted in other terms by Loewenstein, referring to Hartmann, is the avoidance of comprising [sic] by an interpretation, even though accurate, the gradual development of the analysis as a whole. The need for preserving the *rapproacher* in general, is more important than partial interpretation. . . . Thus at a certain moment a simple affirmative will suffice to underline the importance of a destructive phantasy, while its interpretation in the transference would not be well tolerated. [Bouvet 1958, pp. 215–216]

Here we see the conceptual overlap between optimal distance and the use of "tact" (Loewenstein 1951, Poland 1975) in the analytic situation—that intuitive and subtle understanding of every moment of drift of the analysis, and the response that is called for.

Finally, the concept of distance deepens our understanding of certain instances of negative therapeutic reaction. As is well known, Freud (1923) originally considered it a response to "a sense of guilt, which is finding its satisfaction in the illness and refuses to give up the punishment of suffering" (p. 49). The following year, he modified the concept to "a need for punishment" (1924, p. 166) and traced this need to the fantasized oedipal crimes of incest and parricide. Later observers, however, began to discern that more pernicious negative therapeutic reactions are often based on unresolved pre-oedipal issues including (a) a feeling of guilt in having a separate existence or "separation guilt" (Modell 1965) and (b) a characterological defense against the dread of symbiotic fusion (Asch 1976). A narcissistically needy mother who cannot let go of her child renders him vulnerable to unconsciously equating separation with causing injury to her, even killing her. Asch (1976) notes that certain "specific accusations by mother (your birth was so difficult, I almost died; I was so torn up inside) often add fixating elements of historical 'reality' " (p. 392) to such fears. Subsequent separations, as heralded by any increase in distance (at first from the primary objects and later from their transferential recreations), provoke guilt and are dreaded. Besides Modell (1965) and Asch (1976), Gruenert (1979) has noted negative therapeutic reactions based upon guilt and anxiety of separation. I too have briefly commented elsewhere (Akhtar 1991) on a patient who, with each progressive movement in her analysis, would develop a fear of abandonment by me and, motivated by this fear, a regressive loss of her newly acquired insights.[10]

The second dynamic mentioned above derives from the negativism of oral and anal conflicts that is used to guard against oral fusion or anal submission fantasies. Here compliance with the analyst, especially that based upon a recognition of the validity of his stance, stirs up the dread of symbiotic fusion and a threat to the integrity of the self (Asch 1976). While I have some reservation in labeling this second phenomenon negative therapeutic reaction, I cannot but note that the issue in both these dynamics is one of distance. In separation guilt the anxiety is about too much distance, and in the defense against fusion dynamic the anxiety is about too little. The analyst's awareness of these concerns would enhance his empathy, modulate his

---

10. Miller (1965) suggests that the exacerbation of symptoms during the terminal phase of analysis might also reflect a defense against separation anxiety.

technique, and minimize such reversals of hard-won battles against other resistances.

SUMMARY

In this chapter I discussed the concept of "optimal distance," noting that a dialectical tension between the interpersonal and intrapsychic perspectives is essential to its proper definition. I described the gross psychopathology of optimal distance, including various types of severe character pathology, neurotic formations such as agoraphobia, and certain fluctuating marital difficulties. Following this, I highlighted the more subtle anxieties in this realm and described the tether fantasy and its variants involving orbits and invisible fences. I then reviewed the development of optimal distance and its disturbances. I also attempted to show the reverberations of these phenomena in the sociocultural realm of childhood games, thrill seeking, travel, vacations, migration, and exile. Finally, I devoted a lengthier section of the chapter to the varied and profound implications of these concepts to the technique of psychoanalysis and intensive psychotherapy.

Let me conclude with two disclaimers. First, although I have emphasized the pre-oedipal basis for the development of optimal distance and its pathology, this should not be taken to mean that I do not recognize the oedipal contributions to these matters. Indeed, I have mentioned them briefly in this chapter. Second, with the exception of my description of the tether fantasy and its variants, I do not claim any significant originality to ideas presented here. My work has largely been one of synthesis and exposition. Through this, I have attempted to extend the work of many outstanding analysts, especially Maurice Bouvet, Michael Balint, and Margaret Mahler.

REFERENCES

Abraham, K. (1913). A constitutional basis of locomotor anxiety. In *Selected Papers of Karl Abraham, M.D.,* pp. 235–244. London: Hogarth Press, 1927.

Adler, G. (1981). The borderline-narcissistic personality disorder continuum. *American Journal of Psychiatry* 138:46-50.

Akhtar, S. (1987). Schizoid personality disorder: a synthesis of developmental, dynamic, and descriptive features. *American Journal of Psychotherapy* 41:499-518.

—— (1988). Hypomanic personality disorder. *Integrative Psychiatry* 6:37-46.

—— (1989). Narcissistic personality disorder: descriptive features and differential diagnosis. *Psychiatric Clinics of North America* 12:505-528.

—— (1990a). Paranoid personality disorder: a synthesis of developmental, dynamic, and descriptive features. *American Journal of Psychotherapy* 44:5-25.

—— (1990b). Concept of interpersonal distance in borderline personality disorder. *American Journal of Psychiatry* 147:260-261.

—— (1991). Three fantasies related to unresolved separation-individuation: a less recognized aspect of severe character pathology. In *Beyond the Symbiotic Orbit: Advances in Separation-Individuation Theory,* ed. S. Akhtar and H. Parens, pp. 261-284. Hillsdale, NJ: The Analytic Press.

Asch, S. (1976). Varieties of negative therapeutic reaction and problems of technique. *Journal of the American Psychoanalytic Association* 24:383-407.

Bach, S. (1985). The narcissistic state of consciousness. In *Narcissistic States and the Therapeutic Process,* pp. 3-47. New York: Jason Aronson.

Balint, M. (1959). *Thrills and Regression.* London: Hogarth Press.

Bergman, A. (1980). Ours, yours, mine. In *Rapprochement: The Critical Subphase of Separation-Individuation,* ed. R. Lax, S. Bach, and J. A. Burland, pp. 199-216. New York: Jason Aronson.

Blos, P. (1967). The second individuation process of adolescence. *Psychoanalytic Study of the Child* 22:162-186. New York: International Universities Press.

Blum, H. (1981). Object constancy and paranoid conspiracy. *Journal of the American Psychoanalytic Association* 29:789-813.

Bouvet, M. (1958). Technical variation and the concept of distance. *International Journal of Psycho-Analysis* 39:211-221.

Boyer, (1967). Office treatment of schizophrenic patients: the use of psychoanalytic therapy with few parameters. In *Psychoanalytic Treatment of Characterological and Schizophrenic Disorders,* ed. L. B. Boyer and P. L. Giovacchini, pp. 143-188. New York: Science House.

Burland, A. J. (1975). Separation-individuation and reconstruction in psychoanalysis. *International Journal of Psychoanalytic Psychotherapy* 4:303-335.

Burnham, D. L., Gladstone, A. E., and Gibson, R. W. (1969). *Schizophrenia and the Need-Fear Dilemma.* New York: International Universities Press.

Chmiel, A. J., Akhtar, S., and Morris, J. (1979). The long-distance psychiatric patient in the emergency room: insights regarding travel and mental illness. *International Journal of Social Psychiatry* 25:38-46.

Cirlot, J. E. (1971). *A Dictionary of Symbols.* Trans. J. Sage. New York: Philosophical Library.

Deutsch, F. (1952). Analytic posturology. *Psychoanalytic Quarterly* 21:196-214.

Deutsch, H. (1929). The genesis of agoraphobia. *International Journal of Psycho-Analysis* 10:51-69.

——— (1942). Some forms of emotional disturbance and their relationship to schizophrenia. *Psychoanalytic Quarterly* 11:301-321.
Dewall, R. (1984). *Korczak: Storyteller in Stone.* Crazy Horse, SD: Korczak's Heritage.
Erikson, E. (1950). *Childhood and Society.* New York: W. W. Norton.
Fairbairn, W. R. D. (1952). *An Object-Relations Theory of the Personality.* New York: Basic Books.
Fenichel, O. (1945). *The Psychoanalytic Theory of Neurosis.* New York: W. W. Norton.
Fischer, N. (1991). *The psychoanalytic experience and psychic change.* Paper presented at the 27th biannual meeting of the International Psychoanalytical Association, Buenos Aires, Argentina, August.
Frank, A. (1969). The unrememberable and the unforgettable: passive primal repression. *Psychoanalytic Study of the Child* 24:48-77. New York: International Universities Press.
Freud, A. (1936). *The Ego and the Mechanisms of Defense.* New York: International Universities Press.
Freud, S. (1892-1899). Extracts from the Fleiss papers. *Standard Edition* 1:173-280.
——— (1893-1895). Studies on hysteria (with J. Breuer). *Standard Edition* 2:1-323.
——— (1905). The psychopathology of everyday life. *Standard Edition* 6:1-310.
——— (1910). A special type of choice of object made by men. *Standard Edition* 11:163-176.
——— (1915a). Instincts and their vicissitudes. *Standard Edition* 14:110-140.
——— (1915b). The unconscious. *Standard Edition* 14:159-216.
——— (1920). Beyond the pleasure principle. *Standard Edition* 18:7-64.
——— (1921). Group psychology and the analysis of the ego. *Standard Edition* 18:67-144.
——— (1923). The ego and the id. *Standard Edition* 17:12-68.
——— (1924). The dissolution of the oedipus complex. *Standard Edition* 19:171-188.
——— (1926). Inhibitions, symptoms and anxiety. *Standard Edition* 20:77-174.
Gediman, H. K. (1985). Imposture, inauthenticity and feeling fraudulent. *Journal of the American Psychoanalytic Association* 33:911-936.
Gibran, K. (1923). *The Prophet.* New York: Alfred A. Knopf.
Glenn, G. (1991). Transformation in normal and pathological latency. In *Beyond the Symbiotic Orbit: Advances in Separation-Individuation Theory—Essays in Honor of Selma Kramer, M.D.,* ed. S. Akhtar and H. Parens, pp. 171-187. Hillsdale, NJ: The Analytic Press.
Greenacre, P. (1953). Certain relationships between fetishism and the faulty development of the body image. *Psychoanalytic Study of the Child* 8:79-97. New York: International Universities Press.
Grinberg, L. R., and Grinberg, R. (1984). A psychoanalytic study of migration: its normal and pathological aspects. *Journal of the American Psychoanalytic Association* 32:13-38.
——— (1989). *Psychoanalytic Perspectives on Migration and Exile.* New Haven: Yale University Press.
Grinstein, A. (1955). Vacations: a psycho-analytic study. *International Journal of Psycho-Analysis* 36:177-186.

Gruenert, U. (1979). The negative therapeutic reaction as a reactivation of a disturbed process of separation in the transference. *Bulletin of European Psychoanalytical Federation* 16:5-19.

Gunderson, J. (1985). *Borderline Personality Disorder.* Washington, DC: American Psychiatric Press.

Guntrip, H. (1969). *Schizoid Phenomena, Object Relations and the Self.* New York: International Universities Press.

——— (1975). My experience of analysis with Fairbairn and Winnicott. *International Review of Psycho-Analysis* 2:145-156.

Guttman, S. A., Jones, R. L., and Parrish, S. M., eds. (1980). *The Concordance to the Standard Edition of the Complete Psychological Works of Sigmund Freud,* vol. 2, p. 203. Boston: G. K. Hall.

Hinsie, L. E. and Campbell, R. J. (1975). *Psychiatric Dictionary.* 4th ed. New York: Oxford University Press.

Kaplan, Z. (1971). Eruv. In *Encyclopedia Judaica,* vol. 6, p. 849. Jerusalem: Keter Publishing House.

Kernberg, O. F. (1970). Factors in the psychoanalytic treatment of narcissistic personalities. *Journal of the American Psychoanalytic Association* 18:51-85.

Klauber, J. (1971). Personal attitudes to psychoanalytic consultation. In *Difficulties in the Analytic Encounter,* pp. 141-159. New York: Jason Aronson, 1981.

Kleeman, J. A. (1967). The peek-a-boo game, part 1: its origins, meanings, and related phenomena in the first year. *Psychoanalytic Study of the Child* 22:239-273. New York: International Universities Press.

Kohut, H. (1980). Summarizing reflections. In *Advances in Self Psychology,* ed. A. Goldberg, pp. 473-554. New York: International Universities Press.

Laplanche, J. and Pontalis, J. B. (1973). *The Language of Psycho-Analysis.* Trans. D. Nicholson-Smith. New York: Norton.

Loewenstein, R. (1951). The problem of interpretation. *Psychoanalytic Quarterly* 20:1-23.

Mahler, M. S. (1965). On the significance of the normal separation–individuation phase with reference to research in symbiotic childhood psychosis. In *The Selected Papers of Margaret S. Mahler,* vol. 2, pp. 49-58. New York: Jason Aronson.

——— (1971). A study of the separation–individuation process and its possible application to borderline phenomena in the psychoanalytic situation. In *The Selected Papers of Margaret S. Mahler,* vol. 2, pp. 169-187. New York: Jason Aronson.

——— (1972). On the first three subphases of the separation–individuation process. In *The Selected Papers of Margaret S. Mahler,* vol. 2, pp. 119-130. New York: Jason Aronson.

——— (1974). Symbiosis and individuation: the psychological birth of the human infant. In *The Selected Papers of Margaret S. Mahler,* vol. 2, pp. 149-165. New York: Jason Aronson.

——— (1975). On the current status of the infantile neurosis. In *Selected Papers of Margaret S. Mahler,* vol. 2, pp. 189-193. New York: Jason Aronson.

Mahler, M. S., Pine, F., and Bergman, A. (1975). *The Psychological Birth of the Infant.* New York: Basic Books.

Melges, F. T., and Swartz, M. S. (1989). Oscillations of attachment in borderline personality disorder. *American Journal of Psychiatry* 146:1115–1120.
Miller, J. (1965). On the return of symptoms in the terminal phase of psychoanalysis. *International Journal of Psycho-Analysis* 46:487–501.
Mittleman, B. (1957). Motility in the therapy of children and adults. *Psychoanalytic Study of the Child* 12:284–319. New York: International Universities Press.
Modell, A. (1965). On aspects of the superego's development. *International Journal of Psycho-Analysis* 46:323–331.
——— (1984). *Psychoanalysis in a New Context.* New York: International Universities Press.
Moore, B. E., and Fine, B. D., eds. (1968). *A Glossary of Psychoanalytic Terms and Concepts.* New York: American Psychoanalytic Association.
——— (1990). *Psychoanalytic Terms and Concepts.* New Haven: Yale University Press.
Phillips, R. H. (1960). The nature and function of children's formal games. *Psychoanalytic Quarterly* 29:200–207.
Poland, W. S. (1975). Tact as a psychoanalytic function. *International Journal of Psycho-Analysis* 56:155.
——— (1977). Pilgrimage: action and tradition in self-analysis. *Journal of the American Psychoanalytic Association* 25(2):399–416.
Pollock, G. (1989). On migration—voluntary and coerced. *The Annual of Psychoanalysis* 17:145–619.
Pruett, K. D. (1990). *The impact of involved fatherhood on child development: research and clinical perspectives.* Paper presented at the meeting of the Philadelphia Psychoanalytic Society, October.
A Psychiatric Glossary (1975). Washington, DC: American Psychiatric Association.
Rossner, J. (1983). *August.* Boston: Houghton Mifflin.
Roth, M. (1959). The phobic anxiety depersonalization syndrome. *Proceedings of the Royal Society of Medicine* 52:587–595.
Rycroft, C. (1972). *A Critical Dictionary of Psychoanalysis.* London: Penguin Books.
Sandler, J. (1987). Internalization and externalization. In *Projection, Identification and Projective Identification,* ed. J. Sandler, pp. 1–12. Madison, CT: International Universities Press.
Schopenhauer, A. (1981). *The Pessimist's Handbook: A Collection of Popular Essays.* Trans. T. B. Sauders, ed. H. E. Barnes. Omaha: University of Nebraska Press.
Spitz, R. (1965). *The First Year of Life.* New York: International Universities Press.
Sterba, E. (1940). Homesickness and the mother's breast. *Psychiatric Quarterly* 14:701–707.
Strachey, J. (1934). The nature of the therapeutic action of psychoanalysis. *International Journal of Psycho-Analysis* 15:127–159.
Teja, J. S., and Akhtar, S. (1981). The psycho-social problems of FMGs with special references to those in psychiatry. In *Foreign Medical Graduates in Psychiatry: Issues and Problems,* ed. R. S. Chen, pp. 321–338. New York: Human Sciences Press.
Volkan, V. D. (1987). *Six Steps in the Treatment of Borderline Personality Disorder.* Northvale, NJ: Jason Aronson.

Volkan, V. D., and Corney, R. T. (1968). Some considerations of satellite states and satellite dreams. *British Journal of Medical Psychology* 41:283-290.

Waelder, R. (1933). The psychoanalytic theory of play. *Psychiatric Quarterly* 2:208.

——— (1930). The principle of multiple function: observations on multiple determination. *Psychoanalytic Quarterly* 5:45-62.

Warren, M. (1961). The significance of visual images during the analytic session. *Journal of the Ameican Psychoanalytic Association* 9:504-518.

Weiss, E. (1964). *Agoraphobia in the Light of Ego Psychology*. New York: Grune and Stratton.

Wheelis, A. (1966). *The Illusionless Man*. New York: Colophon Books/Harper & Row.

Winnicott, D. W. (1953). Transitional objects and transitional phenomena: a study of the first not-me possession. *International Journal of Psycho-Analysis* 34:89-97.

——— (1960a). String: a technique of communication. In *The Maturational Process and the Facilitating Environment*, pp. 153-157. New York: International Universities Press.

——— (1960b). The theory of the parent–infant relationship. *International Journal of Psycho-Analysis* 41:585-595.

——— (1971). *Playing and Reality*. New York: Basic Books.

3

VICISSITUDES OF OPTIMAL DISTANCE THROUGH THE LIFE CYCLE

Discussion of Akhtar's Chapter, "Tethers, Orbits, and Invisible Fences: Clinical, Developmental, Sociocultural, and Technical Aspects of Optimal Distance"

Philip J. Escoll, M.D.

Dr. Salman Akhtar brings the concept of optimal distance out of the shadows of psychoanalytic discourse and into the open for a consideration of its meaning, significance, and application to a variety of important areas. Dr. Akhtar begins by noting Freud's emphasis on the body and the somatic underpinnings of his theories. He reviews Balint's (1959) work and cites Bouvet (1958) and Mahler (1971, 1975) as defining optimal distance in the interpersonal and in the intrapsychic spheres. He reviews Mahler's symbiotic and separation–individuation stages as they relate to the concept of optimal distance. He states that "if the mother is not optimally available during the rapprochement subphase, the contradictory self and object representations remain split and capacity for optimal distance fails to develop. This leads to a lifelong tendency toward oscillations between passionate intimacy and hateful withdrawal from objects." He goes on to say that "in light of this, 'optimal distance' is best viewed as a psychic position which permits intimacy without loss of autonomy, and separateness without painful aloneness."

Dr. Akhtar then discusses the psychopathology of optimal distance; he considers agoraphobia, claustrophobia and severe personality disorders from this standpoint. He turns to fantasies, the tether fantasy and others, as examples of fantasies employed to deal with conflicts related to optimal distance, which emerge in the course of adult analyses. Dr. Akhtar then considers the sociocultural vicissitudes of optimal distance in childhood games, travel and vacations, immigration and exile. In conclusion, Dr. Akhtar discusses the technical implications of the concept of distance in analysis. He gives examples from analytic work of the need for analyst and patient to maintain optimal distance. He emphasizes that it "remains the analyst's responsibility to safeguard this optimal distance."

In my discussion of his chapter, I first comment on the definition and vicissitudes of optimal distance. Then I offer some illustrations of animal behavior, along with works of art, to provide a graphic demonstration of the bodily expressions of optimal distance. I also cite a few examples from fiction and poetry alluding to conflicts about optimal distance. Finally, I describe an analytic case and consider the application of this concept to the analytic process.

THE CONCEPT OF OPTIMAL DISTANCE

Psychoanalysis began with the body. In his "Project for a Scientific Psychology," Freud (1895) saw the intimate connection between mind and body as the "mainspring of the psychical mechanism" (p. 316). His early emphasis on constitution, the body ego, and actual neurosis, his belief in the economic theory (quantities of energy), and his conviction that hormonal and chemical processes were the underpinning of the psyche attest to this.

Physicians have always felt that the laying on of hands was vital in the treatment of patients. Freud, as part of his hypnotic technique in the early days of experimentation with psychoanalysis, would place his hand on the patient's forehead. As Stewart (1989) describes, Balint would at times hold the patient's finger or hand.

We are well aware of the importance of tactile sensations to the infant and child (Barnard and Brazelton 1990), as well as the significance of being held and cuddled to the adult (Hollander 1970). Of course, "touching" is also provided with sensations and experiences other than tactile ones, such as eye contact, taste, smell, and voice. What does this have to do with optimal distance? I believe it illustrates the importance of bodily sensations in regard to the separation–individuation process and, therefore, to optimal distance. Being held, moving away, looking back, listening for mother's voice, climbing into mother's lap, touching her face, being hugged, and hugging back are all part of the process, as Mahler and colleagues (1975) certainly understood. How close to or how far from another body or person an individual needs to be to secure comfortable optimal distance is influenced by bodily sensations and experiences.

I agree with Dr. Akhtar that optimal distance reflects both interpersonal and intrapsychic components. It is expressed in the interpersonal sphere and definitely has its bodily manifestations. Of course, it also has its intrapsychic representations related to self and object, or self-object. Bouvet is credited, I believe, with originating the term in his 1958 paper. Mahler's descriptions of separation–individuation phases, with the crucible of rapprochement, and the "eternal struggle against both fusion and isolation" (Mahler 1972, p. 130) are fundamental to our understanding of optimal distance. In his description of the dilemma of the schizoid individual, Guntrip (1969) also used similar ideas. Object constancy is a related concept of significance in the establishment of optimal distance. Erikson's (1950, 1968) concepts of intimacy and isolation and identity diffusion also apply, especially to the adolescent and young adult.

Why do we use the term "optimal distance" and not "optimal closeness"? Edward and colleagues (1981) use the latter term in their work. Perhaps there is a gender difference involved, in that males strive for independence and distance while females seek relatedness and closeness (Gilligan 1982). These gender-determined differences begin in childhood and persist throughout adult life. They also have an impact on parenting attitudes in certain situations. Pruett (1990) explored the possibility, for example, that the father permits the child in play to go farther away than the mother does.

The concept of optimal distance may be employed in either a narrow or a broad fashion. Dr. Akhtar employs the concept broadly, and, as with any concept, there are advantages and disadvantages to this. I think we lose something if we use the concept too broadly, diverging from the Mahlerian meaning of the term. Of course, as with any explanatory concept, we need to be mindful of how we are defining it and of all the forces involved, following Waelder's (1930) principle of multiple function. In thinking about optimal-distance conflicts in personality disorders and other clinical entities, problems with intimacy and closeness, and difficulties related to sexuality and aggression, we also need to consider the influence and power of multiple motivations, of unconscious fantasies and defense mechanisms, and, in treatment, of transference and countertransference factors.

There are many related questions one can raise about optimal distance. Arriving at an optimal distance has to do with how well one has resolved the separation–individuation phases, particularly the practicing and rapprochement phases, and the requisite maternal availability that is necessary in those phases. The role of the father is also of great importance in establishing optimal distance, and this should not be overlooked as it too often is. It is the father who can aid and facilitate appropriate distancing from the mother in the symbiotic and separation–individuation phases. Further, one could ask what leads one person to establish an optimal distance intrapsychically, with its interpersonal manifestations, that is relatively close and another to establish great distance. Does the use of a transitional object influence the achievement of optimal distance?

One person's distance may be another person's closeness. Also, while physical distance/closeness is certainly important, it is not necessarily the same as emotional closeness. Characterological optimal distances are also influenced by constitutional and cultural factors. The concept of optimal distance has its pragmatic applications: speak to an engineer as he is calibrating the appropriate size of an elevator to provide sufficient private space for each individual, also the engineer planning the space between seats in an auditorium—not too close to make people uncomfortable, not too distant.

In the separation–individuation phase, the child establishes optimal distance but the parents also establish their optimal distance from the child. Obviously, parents need to respond to the particular needs of the individual child, but they must also be responsive to their own background and needs. To paraphrase Kegan (1982), parents need to hold on, let go, stick around. Optimal distance has its vicissitudes for parents as well as for children.

Some difficulty with distance/closeness occurs in a wide variety of individuals across the spectrum of emotional disorders and character types. Ideally, one can achieve an optimal distance that oscillates comfortably depending on the degree of object attachment as well as internal factors, one's mood, fantasies, and so on. Some people have a fixed optimal distance, which has little flexibility and is maintained under almost any circumstance. A psychotherapy patient of mine seemed to have an invisible ruler, because she noted with alarm whenever her chair had been moved even a fraction of an inch. She would become irritated and agitated and immediately push the chair so that it would be in exactly the right position for her; leaning forward or backward in the chair, as many do, was not enough. Incidentally, the psychotherapy chair that my patients use is on rollers. I cannot

claim that I selected the chair on rollers to facilitate optimal distance—it was probably on sale.

Optimal distance and its vicissitudes, like the reverberations of separation–individuation, are seen through the life cycle. For example, going away to camp or college or moving to another city may produce the syndrome of homesickness. Gould (1978) writes of the experience of children owning their own homes for the first time: "A tether to our parents was torn, and we mourned it. We were a bit less fettered by the codes of life our parents had woven in to the tether, but we were left temporarily unanchored in time and space" (p. 11).

The syndrome of homesickness relates to being away from home, from home base, with the wish to return or know that one may return. There is something important in the degree of distance. The individual is often more comfortable beginning with the college or camp in the same state or closer to home than in a distant place.

Death is the final parting from home and from the people with whom the individual is connected. Egyptians dealt with this by sending familiar objects and servants along on the journey of the dead to the underworld. In Anne Tyler's *The Accidental Tourist* (1985), the travel writer makes sure that he packs all of the necessary ingredients of his home environment; in his books he advises Americans where they can go to get hamburgers, English-language newspapers, and other artifacts of home when they are abroad.

OPTIMAL DISTANCE, SEXUALITY, AND AGGRESSION

Issues of optimal distance are also an important factor in clinical problems related to sexuality and aggression. Here the internal bodily representations of self and object are of tremendous significance. Men may fear engulfment by women: some male patients describe the vagina as a vast cavern, a cave, and have a fearful fantasy of being permanently lost or imprisoned in it. To defend against this, emotional and/or physical distance is established. In turn, women frequently complain that there is too much distance on the male's part and insufficient cuddling or hugging, particularly as related to sexuality.

There are related forces at work regarding aggression. Distance may be stretched, for example, to avoid the dangerous expression of one's own aggressive impulses or to avoid retaliation. Distancing may also be used to express contempt and anger. This may be done by physically distancing oneself and becoming emotionally remote through inattentiveness, detachment, and silence. On the other hand, closeness may express aggression with such reactions as a crushing embrace or a fracturing handshake. Excessive closeness may express aggression, as with the baseball manager arguing with the umpire by putting his face into the umpire's and kicking dirt at him. Anger may be avoided by a false kind of closeness, such as hugging or kissing to pacify a partner and disguise the individual's hostility. In all of these situations played out bodily and interpersonally there are, of course, intrapsychic conflicts, including those that involve the self and object representations in optimal distance.

The issue of boundaries has many dimensions but may be related to optimal distance. Transgressions of boundaries and abrogation of optimal distance in situations involving rape and sexual and physical abuse are of far-reaching significance. These transgressions carry ramifications that may lead to dissociative and posttraumatic stress disorders and may contribute to borderline personalities.

There is also the necessary "transgression" of boundaries involving romantic sexual stimulation and excitement. Overcoming the oedipal barrier, Kernberg (1976) says, is part of the love relation for men and women. The relationships in dating, courtship, and marriage bring out issues of optimal distance. Couples who get along well obviously work out their own particular arrangement of optimal distance. Others seem to be constantly quarreling about matters that may be derivatives of the optimal distance issue—who has pulled the covers to whose side, for example, or what size bed to have, a queen or a king. Some couples establish their variety of optimal distance by living apart. Woody Allen and Mia Farrow, for example, as described by Lax (1991), live in different apartment buildings and communicate with each other by waving towels outside their respective windows.

THE TETHER FANTASY

Dr. Akhtar makes very interesting reference to tether and related fantasies, such as being in an orbit. It is not unusual in my experience for patients to have fantasies of being in orbit both figuratively and literally. There is the fantasy of being in a spaceship establishing distance from earth and home base, yet maintaining connection by being in orbit. Some patients fantasize about taking the analyst along on the journey (Fischer 1991). In his section on the tether fantasy, Dr. Akhtar cites Freud's (1920) description of his grandson and the wooden reel and Winnicott's (1960) patient, a 7-year-old boy, who was preoccupied with tying household objects together with string. In *Celestial Navigation* (1974), Anne Tyler gives a wonderful description of a man completely tied to his mother:

> If he tried to conquer the very worst of his dreads—set out on a walk, for instance, ignoring the strings that stretched so painfully between home and the center of his back—his legs first became extremely heavy so that every movement was a great aching effort, and then his heart started pounding and his breath grew shallow and he felt nauseated. If he succeeded in spite of everything, in finishing what he had set out to do, he had no feeling of accomplishment but only a trembling weakness, like someone

recently brushed by danger and an echo of the nausea and a deep sense of despair. He took no steps forward. [p. 77]

The tether fantasy raises the question of umbilical cord fantasies. These may exist in direct forms as well as in displaced and derivative forms, but I have not heard the direct umbilical cord fantasy from a patient. One substitute for this in action as well as in fantasy is the telephone, which often serves as a tether, an umbilical cord. The telephone obviously provides a connection, also a separation, particularly when it doesn't ring. An analytic patient of mine moved from city to city and country to country with her father, who worked in the diplomatic service. She remembers his calling from faraway places when she was little, and also remembers times when he could not call and there would be no communication for a period of time. Her pattern in her young adult life with her boyfriends has been to wait expectantly and anxiously for their calls and to literally, physically cling to the phone at these times. In her fantasies, attachment would be sustained or severed by the telephone. If boyfriends did not call, as she expected them to, she would experience great anxiety and then a deep feeling of abandonment. Once, when she expected someone she had recently started to date to call and he did not, she became so anxious and so fearful that the only way she could deal with it was to call him in a rage and tell him she would never see him again. Early in the analysis she also would call my answering machine at night, not so much to leave a message as to have contact with me through my recorded voice. This would reassure her, and she would be able to wait for the next appointment.

Disregarding the boundary or casting off the attaching tether leads to a sense of thrill, as Balint (1959) has described in the person with "philobatic" attitudes. There are those who require the security of a tether to home; on the other side, there are those who enjoy being away from home base and throwing off the symbolic tether. This is true in regard to travel but is also seen in activities (e.g., parachute jumping, hang gliding, skiing) often described as "thrilling" and giving one a sense of "being free" or "with the elements." Such physical considerations lead me to a further, though brief, digression into certain other realms.

ANIMALS, ART, AND LITERATURE

In this section, I demonstrate the bodily expressions of optimal distance in animal behavior. I also provide a few examples from art and literature.

Animal Kingdom

Ethological observations disclose related patterns of maintaining optimal distance in animal behavior. For example, in many species the young are assigned a very definite prescribed orbit by the mother beyond which they do not go. This raises the question of constitutional, genetic, and species-specific elements in optimal distance. Of course, in discussing animals I am using optimal distance in a very concrete sense, not as we conceptualize the term; obviously, animals do not have the intrapsychic representations of self and object that humans do. Most of all, I am using the following animal examples to provide graphic corporeal illustrations of optimal distance.

Illustration 1. In this photograph, two adult giraffes are seen with their very long necks intertwined, but not touching. Here, their own version of corporeal optimal distance is seen in the intimacy of the linkage of the necks and yet the very definite posture of not touching each other.

Illustration 2. Optimal distance in a very literal sense is seen here. The mother elephant's body is close enough to protect

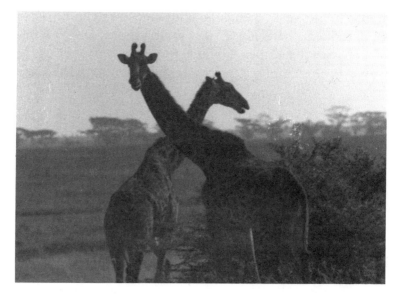

Illustration #1, Philip J. Escoll, M.D., East Africa

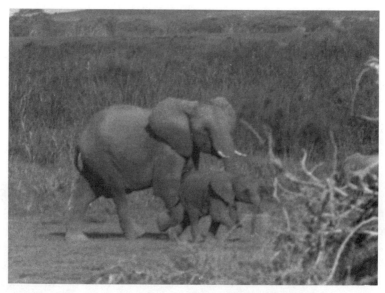

Illustration #2, Philip J. Escoll, M.D., East Africa

Vicissitudes of Optimal Distance Through the Life Cycle

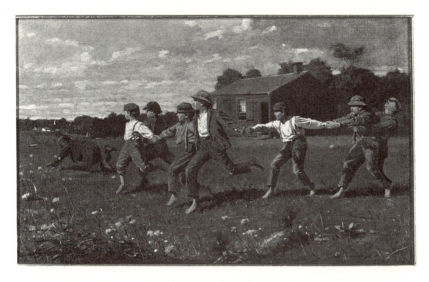

Illustration #3, *Snap the Whip,* Winslow Homer. Courtesy of the Metropolitan Museum of Art, Gift of Christian A. Zabriskie, 1950. (50.41).

but distant enough not to harm her offspring. Optimal distance must be maintained scrupulously for survival.

Paintings

The nineteenth-century American painter Winslow Homer was known as a reclusive bachelor in the small town in Maine where he spent his later years. However, in the town he was known as a very friendly person who always stopped to greet passersby and chat with them. He seemed to have little trouble in establishing brief connections, but longer-lasting ones were difficult for him (Beam 1966, Prown 1987).

Illustration 3. *Snap the Whip* by Winslow Homer. In this painting, boys are playing a game called snap the whip, which has to do with both connection and disconnection, closeness and distance. The object of the game is to break the linkage by

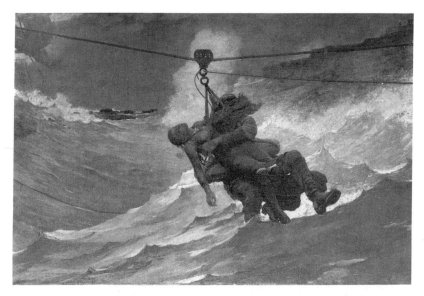

Illustration #4, *The Life Line,* Winslow Homer. Courtesy of the Philadelphia Museum of Art, George W. Elkins Collection.

propelling the boys apart while at the same time striving to stay together by holding hands as tightly as possible. The artist has conveyed a psychological distance as well, in that the boys do not look at one another.

Illustration 4. *The Life Line* by Winslow Homer. This painting of a rescue at sea shows a man and woman clinging to each other and to a tether, a line that connects them to life. Note, however, that although they are holding on to one another, there is a separation between them created by a life preserver. The intensity of their connection is motivated by survival and seems to have erotic connotations.

Illustration 5. *The Gulf Stream* by Winslow Homer. This painting brings out the aloneness, isolation, and resignation of a man adrift at sea. He is also in great danger; his boat is demasted

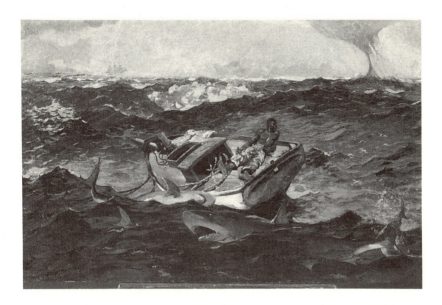

Illustration #5, *The Gulf Stream,* Winslow Homer. Courtesy of the Metropolitan Museum of Art, Wolfe Fund, 1906. Catherine Lorillard Wolfe Collection. (06.1234)

and nonfunctional, and he is surrounded by sharks and turbulent waters. No human attachment is present; optimal distance is fractured. This work is the antithesis of the attachment in *Snap the Whip* and the couple's desperate clutching of each other and the tether in *The Life Line*.

Sculpture

Illustration 6. *The Kiss* by Constantin Brancusi. The optimal distance is obvious in this piece. Here Brancusi expresses the absolute union of the male and female figures. They are portrayed with solidity and compactness; they are exactly the same size, locked together, virtually fused, in their erotic embrace. Brancusi had his own struggles with optimal distance.

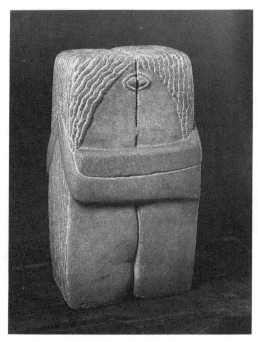

Illustration #6, *The Kiss,* Constantin Brancusi. Courtesy of the Philadelphia Museum of Art, Louise and Walter Arensberg Collection.

Reared in Romania, he reputedly left his home at age 11 and walked from the small village in which he lived to another town. Subsequently, as a young adult, it is said that he walked from Romania to Paris.

Fiction

Literature is filled with references that relate to the concept of optimal distance. For example, in the legend of the Flying Dutchman the captain must remain on his boat as punishment for blasphemy, although he must come to land every seven years. In E. E. Hale's *The Man Without a Country,* the protagonist has renounced his citizenship and is permanently exiled with no country available to him. These characters are figuratively and literally at sea, painfully distanced from home base. Their tethers have been virtually severed. Odysseus, on the other hand, leaves home and wanders for years, but at the same time his attachment remains constant because he is determined to return to his wife, Penelope. At one point he asks his sailors to tether him to the mast so that he will not heed the call of the sirens. Anne Tyler often uses the theme of optimal distance in her novels; this is especially true in *Celestial Navigation* (1974) and *The Accidental Tourist* (1985).

Virginia Woolf, who lost her mother in her youth, describes a search for a lighthouse in her novel, *To the Lighthouse* (1927). While there are multiple motivations involved, including looking for a phallic symbol, one can also see the search for the lighthouse as the search for closeness with the lost mother. Handelman (1980) states that *To the Lighthouse*

> deals with the central problem of the disillusion of the symbiotic union of early mother–child relationship and the child's resultant quest for a lost primal unity and yet antithetical drive for independent identity. [p. 48]

The yellow brick road in *The Wizard of Oz* by Frank L. Baum (1900) may be seen as an example of a tether. Dorothy has a dream in which she leaves home and runs away; she tries to recapture her dog, Toto, who may represent a transitional object, and in the dream there are figures from childhood who are transformed. The yellow brick road is her path of moving away from home, but at the same time it provides her with a way to return. When Dorothy reaches Emerald City, she proclaims her wish to go home, to go home to Kansas and Auntie Em. As she awakens from her dream, the mother figure, Auntie Em, is there and Dorothy exclaims in the delight of closeness and reunion, "Auntie Em, Auntie Em."

Poetry

Dr. Akhtar refers to invisible fences as an optimal distance fantasy. Such allusions are not infrequent in poetry. In "The Mending Wall," Robert Frost (1914) takes both sides of the optimal distance equation, that is, the wall as an unnecessary dividing marker between spaces and people and as a necessary and useful barrier. In this poem, the issues of closeness, distance, and boundaries are implied. "He only says, 'good fences make good neighbors' . . . 'why do they make good neighbors? . . . Something there is that doesn't love a wall, that wants it down.'"

After this brief digression into the arts, I now want to return to clinical issues and discuss a patient (see also Escoll 1991) who had great difficulties with optimal distance.

A CLINICAL ILLUSTRATION

Mr. R., a 25-year-old salesman, began analysis depressed and confused about an affair he had begun a year earlier. This young married adult had initially found his involvement with another woman tremendously pleasurable owing to the way he could talk to and be understood by her. This gratification remained primary even as the relationship became sexualized. Complications ensued when his lover became periodically reinvolved with her own husband from whom she had separated. During these periods, Mr. R. began pondering his future with his own wife, alternating between an inclination to leave her and a resolve to strengthen their relationship.

As tension entered the extramarital affair and Mr. R. began to withdraw from his lover, the latter gave mixed signals of her own: she alternated between pleading her devotion and asking Mr. R. to wait for her and announcing that the affair was over and that she was contemplating returning to her husband. Mr. R.

responded to these contradictory messages with confusion and unhappiness, periodically lapsing into depression. He would wait by the phone for his girlfriend to call, feeling enormously relieved when she did, but depressed to the point of tears and hopelessness about his future when she did not.

As we tried to understand these disturbing episodes, Mr. R.'s relationship to his mother during the separation–individuation process assumed major importance. Specifically, Mr. R. associated back to what was probably a rapprochement crisis when he was between the ages of 2 and 3. He recollected his mother's own on again, off again behavior during this time: she could be loving one moment, cold and withdrawn the next. Her sudden recourse to angry silence followed some small act on his part that gave her displeasure. The misdemeanors that got Mr. R. into trouble with his mother were nothing more than phase-appropriate claims for autonomy and the associated use of his budding motor skills to do things around the house. The patient poignantly recalled his sadness and despair when, following some minor mishap, his otherwise attentive mother subjected him to the "silent treatment."

The mother's alternating pattern of engagement and withdrawal persisted into Mr. R.'s young adulthood. He was aware of periods when she was tender and solicitous, but he was equally aware of periods when, displeased with her son, she would withdraw and maintain a stubborn silence, refusing any communication with him. In the present, as in early childhood, it took very little to occasion such maternal displeasure; often it was simply a matter of Mr. R.'s not calling or visiting his mother frequently enough.

What were the derivatives in Mr. R. of his separation–individuation (especially rapprochement) experiences in light of his mother's own difficulties in handling this phase and the associated difficulty she had in maintaining comfortable optimal distance? We see many by-products, such as great ambivalence, splitting, identification with his mother, and the recapitulation of the rapprochement pattern in his young adult years. Mr. R. yearned for closeness, intimacy, and sexuality with his wife but could not sustain it; he periodically withdrew from her, emotionally and physically, culminating in his engaging in an affair. Related to his mother's withdrawal and silent treatment, he was exceedingly sensitive to slights and hurts; he tried to avoid them, and when he encountered them he was terribly injured and withdrew. He could not establish or sustain optimal distance. He also experienced great anger, with wishes to destroy the person whom he saw as hurting him or rejecting him. He was afraid of his own aggression at these times, his murderous fantasies representing a derivative of the devouring fantasies of his childhood. This pattern was seen in his young adult life and also in the analysis.

Mr. R. had difficulty in sustaining emotional ties with friends, his wife, and girlfriends, repetitively moving closer then distancing himself. Yet he remained in the relationship with his lover despite the vicissitudes and rejections, unable to break away, yet unable to come to a resolution involving further intimacy with her. In a recapitulation of his reactions to his rapprochement experiences with his mother when she would withdraw from him, he remained glued to the telephone for hours, waiting for his lover to call. He clung to her using the telephone as his tether. He told her not to call him, but he would feel rejected when she did not. He came to realize that he saw her calls as indications that he was still loved, that lover/mother was not shunning him with the terrible silent treatment and withdrawal. In the face of the withdrawal and silent treatment and scolding, Mr. R. became filled with guilt, feeling he had done something terribly wrong to lover/mother, and suffered anxiety and remorse that he had hurt her. He experienced a great need to undo this, manifested by his urgency to return a telephone call in which he had become angry or reproachful.

Mr. R. felt that he was not truly loved by his mother and, as a result, was filled with hurt and rage. He reenacted his own rapprochement by pushing away his lover/mother; however, he did not do this completely, sending her mixed signals so as to invite a return. Revenge was also a motive. The mixed invitation to return led to an overture on his lover's part, one that he then spurned in retaliation. He assumed his mother's part, enacting it with his lover, whom he identified as himself. In his fantasies his lover became a larger-than-life figure, the very powerful and idealized mother. Mr. R. was very much admired and praised; he experienced his mother as engulfing him with her intense wishes for him to be the "golden boy" in the family. He felt that his mother's expectations of him to be the golden boy were to fulfill her own unfulfilled ambitions. These expectations were intensified by a severe illness sustained by his father, which led the father to use a wheelchair some of the time and to be handicapped in his own work. His father was not able to assist him in attenuating his ambivalent tie to the mother, therefore not facilitating achievement of a stable, optimal distance. Mr. R. was the chosen one and was triumphal yet anxious and guilty in the role of the oedipal victor. He resisted the role of the golden boy yet had to achieve it to maintain love; he resented very much being in this position, one that left him feeling inferior and anxious about abandonment on the one hand if he didn't measure up, and grandiose and guilty on the other.

These same feelings were reexperienced with his lover. Mr. R. felt that he had to measure up to her expectations; at the same time, he resented this and felt a tremendous burden to be powerfully successful in his business. With his lover he would feel terribly rejected and angry, with a sense of loss of his prowess and masculinity if she would hint in periods of withdrawal from him that she might become involved with another man or return to her husband. Mr. R. would also berate himself for having done something wrong to elicit this, thus recapitulating the pattern in his childhood when he would alternate between feeling that he had done nothing wrong to lead to his mother's rebukes and withdrawal and feeling that he had done everything wrong. He resented her yet felt that he warranted his mother's scathing rebukes and periods of emotional withdrawal and silence. This pattern was relived with his lover. In his identification with his mother, the aggressor, Mr. R. treated his lover in this hostile way, and she treated him similarly; to a lesser degree he treated his wife this way as well. Interestingly, Mr. R.'s younger brother was described as a clinging person, ambivalently attached to his parents. His brief marriage, which ended in divorce, was fraught with arguments and punctuated by separations and reunions. He too had major difficulty in achieving optimal distance.

It is obvious that many other dynamic issues are involved in Mr. R.'s problems, character, identifications, and relationships with mother, wife, and lover. There were multifaceted oedipal conflicts as well.

In the analysis, Mr. R. gradually realized that his lover's conflicting signals about their relationship paralleled his mother's erratic behavior. He also came to recognize that the despair and hopelessness that followed his mother's withdrawal were the same feelings that followed his girlfriend's intermittent resolve to leave him and return to her husband. Predictably, this pattern, as well as the rapprochement issues inherent in it, was replayed in the transference. To Mr. R., I was attentive and responsive at certain times and coldly withdrawn at others. The latter perception was typically associated with analytic silence; it tended to supervene when Mr. R. felt that he had said or done something (e.g., cancel a session) for which I might be angry. Transference interpretations and reconstructions were central to Mr. R.'s understanding of his conflicts in this area.

Reconstruction was likewise critical. As we arrived at an understanding of Mr. R.'s interaction with his mother during the separation–individuation process and of the intrapsychic derivatives of this interaction, Mr. R. came to see his lover in a new light. This woman, like Mr. R.'s mother, had difficulties with intimacy and optimal distance, probably associated with her own separation–individuation experiences. Mr. R. saw that she yearned to be intimate with him but withdrew uneasily when such intimacy was realized, urging him to "cool it" until she could be sure about her future plans.

The separation–individuation process also provided a handle for understanding Mr. R.'s use of splitting. He tended to see his wife as the cold, asexual mother and his lover as the warm, sexual mother with whom he could have intimate discussions. In addition to the images of the "good" and "bad" mother as residues of the rapprochement subphase, an additional source of the split related to the "madonna" and "whore" split. Mr. R.'s wife was seen as the asexual madonna and the lover as the fun-loving whore. During periods when he and his lover were estranged, Mr. R. saw himself stuck in the house with the bland, dull, asexual wife-mother, and he was filled with envy of the other "kids" who were outside with the daredevil, fun-loving group engaged in sexual exploits with available girls. The pre-oedipal (madonna) and oedipal (whore) split reinforces the earlier split and contributes to its tenacity.

Mr. R.'s lover functioned as a vehicle by which he could separate from the wife-mother on whom he was still quite dependent, even though the lover herself represented another, more favorable side of his mother. Mr. R. himself was prone to take on his mother's role, especially toward his wife; he would periodically become deeply engaged with her, emotionally and sexually, only to withdraw abruptly at a later date. This pattern was played out on the periodic vacations Mr. R. and his wife took. Vowing to leave his lover, Mr. R. would schedule an extended trip, such as a cruise, during which he and his wife would get along wonderfully. While on the trip, however, he would find himself preoccupied with his lover, and immediately on his return he would call her and become reinvolved.

As the foregoing pattern was worked through genetically, transferentially, and in the context of Mr. R.'s current relational triangle, his view of both his wife and his lover changed dramatically. The former was seen as warmer and more affectionate; the latter, toward whom he continued to have tender feelings, as more troubled and manipulative. These reassessments corresponded to a diminished need to recapitulate with these two women the different aspects of his rapprochement experiences with his mother, that is, a diminished need to split the women, albeit interchangeably, into contemporary versions of the "bad mother" and the "good mother" of the rapprochement subphase. To that extent, Mr. R.'s changed feelings toward them betokened structural personality change. He was able to achieve a much better internal resolution of optimal distance between self and objects. This was also seen interpersonally, especially with his wife and with me in the analysis.

IMPLICATIONS FOR THE ANALYTIC PROCESS

In the analytic process one can see the issue of optimal distance at work in many ways. First, there is the direct physical or literal aspect (i.e., the optimal distance/closeness that the patient physically establishes with the analyst). The analyst also has his optimal distance from the patient. Some patients remain relatively motionless on the couch, but others twist and turn in a bid not only to see the analyst but also to move closer to him or farther away. Some are very reactive to the analyst's movements and use this as an indicator of closeness or distance on the analyst's part. The change from sitting up in the evaluation sessions or in psychotherapy to using the couch and entering into the analysis poses many issues related to optimal distance conflicts (Bernstein 1983, Horwitz, 1990, Levine, 1985). The issue of optimal distance is especially important in work with adolescents and young adults who are very sensitive to intrusion and to distance. Beginning with the evaluation interviews the analyst needs to be very alert to both sides of this equation, maintaining appropriate engagement but not being intrusive (Escoll 1987).

Cooper (1990) describes a case of a very difficult, depressed patient. He states,

> [I]t became clear that the treatment, by provoking closeness to a person that she could not control, was making her worse . . . she complained about my distance from her, the actual number of inches between my chair and the couch was intolerable, that I was determined to flee from her, and that something about her made me hate her. My problem was compounded by my increasing uncertainty that I understood her and by my difficulty in maintaining my own benign feelings. Should I move my chair closer when she asked?

We can also consider related aspects of optimal distance, that is, how emotionally close to the patient and to the material the analyst is. Technical neutrality is a related concept that includes Anna Freud's (1936) idea of the analyst taking a position equidistant from the demands of ego, id, and superego. To what degree is there empathic affective attunement? Most patients welcome this attunement, but some find it very difficult. In these individuals it may induce anxiety about closeness and a fear of being engulfed. When others feel empathic contact is not made, they may express a sense of being distant and sometimes experience this with uncomfortable bodily sensations. One can think of optimal distance being involved in terms of the frequency of the sessions, with some patients being uncomfortable meeting five times a week, needing to establish a zone of distance available to them. I am reminded of one of my first analytic patients, a male graduate student, who, for some time in the opening phase of the analysis, had a need to keep one foot on the floor to establish distance from me and also to make a getaway in case of danger.

Some authors use the term "optimal distance" in regard to interpretations. Loewenstein (1951) writes about optimal distance in regard to interpretations being on the surface or having greater depth. Loewald (1960) uses the word "distance" in stating that the analyst's interpretations give the patient distance from himself, enabling him to understand.

In considering the analytic process, however, one always has to remember that optimal distance is a concept that is influenced by many factors. Here the unconscious fantasies that are at work need to be kept in mind because they as well as transference-countertransference obviously influence the patient's reactions. To broaden this consideration of analytic process and to employ optimal distance broadly, going counter to my earlier reservations about broadening the definition, we can think about the evolution of analysis over the last decade or so. We have moved from the idea of the patient on the couch to be analyzed, with the analyst being the objective, distant observer, to the present position of the analyst as a more closely participating observer with all of his own countertransference attitudes. The participant-observer model suggests less distance, greater closeness on the part of the analyst. For example, aspects of the transference have been emphasized, along with the analyst's role in triggering them (Gill 1982). Empathic engagement and affective attunement, as well as alertness to empathic failures (Schwaber 1981), are seen as vital. Countertransference enactments are also very significant, as Jacobs (1986, 1991) has described. Ideally, there is an oscillation between closeness and distance in terms of emotional intimacy and empathy as well as in terms of closeness and distance from the associative material. In all of these instances, there are aspects of Mahler's optimal distance, but clearly this is but one ingredient involved in a complex process with multiple conflicts, motivations, and body language at work in patient and analyst.

SUMMARY

In this discussion of Dr. Akhtar's chapter on optimal distance I have first briefly reviewed the highlights of his paper. The definition of optimal distance and described its vicissitudes through the life cycle. I examined the tether fantasy and its expression in various forms, such as the use of the telephone, as well as the importance of circumstances in which the tether is cast off. In an attempt to illustrate the significance of the body in optimal distance I presented some examples from animal behavior as well as from art and literature. I provided a case history to illustrate clinical problems with optimal distance stemming from failure to satisfactorily resolve the rapprochement subphase of separation–individuation. In conclusion, optimal distance is seen as a useful concept that needs to be understood not only through its origins in the symbiotic and separation–individuation phases, but also in the context of the multiple forces that subsequently impinge upon it in the unfolding life cycle.

REFERENCES

Balint, M. (1959). *Thrills and Regression.* London: Hogarth Press.
Barnard, K., and Brazelton, T. B., eds. (1990). *Touch: The Foundation of Experience.* Madison, CT: International Universities Press.
Baum, L. (1900). *The Wizard of Oz.* New York: Random House.
Beam, P. (1966). *Winslow Homer at Prout's Neck.* Boston: Little, Brown.
Bernstein, S. (1983). Treatment preparatory to psychoanalysis. *Journal of the American Psychoanalytic Association* 31:363–390.
Bouvet, M. (1958). Technical variation and the concept of distance. *International Journal of Psycho-Analysis* 39:211–221.
Cooper, A. (1990). *Some thoughts on how therapy works.* Paper presented at the meeting of the Philadelphia Association for Psychoanalysis, January.
Edward, J., Ruskin, N., and Turrini, P. (1981). *Separation–individuation Theory and Application.* New York: Gardner Press.
Erikson, E. (1950). *Childhood and Society.* New York: Norton.
——— (1968). *Identity: Youth and Crisis.* New York: Norton.
Escoll, P. (1987). Psychoanalysis of adults: an overview. *Psychoanalytic Inquiry* 7:5–30.
——— (1991). Treatment implications of separation–individuation theory in the analysis of young adults. In *Beyond the Symbiotic Orbit: Advances in Separation–Individuation Theory—Essays in Honor of Selma Kramer, M.D.,* ed. S. Akhtar and H. Parens, pp. 369–387. Hillsdale, NJ: Analytic Press.
Fischer, N. (1991). The psychoanalytic experience and psychic change. Paper presented at the 27th biannual meeting of the International Psychoanalytic Association, Buenos Aires, Argentina, August.
Freud, A. (1936). *The Ego and Mechanisms of Defense.* London: Hogarth Press.
Freud, S. (1895). Project for a Scientific Psychology. *Standard Edition* 1:281–397.
——— (1920). Beyond the pleasure principle. *Standard Edition* 17:12–68.
Frost, R. (1914). *Robert Frost's Poems.* New York: Washington Square Press/Pocket Books, 1971.
Gill, M. (1982). *Analysis of Transference/Volume I: Theory and Technique.* New York: International Universities Press.
Gilligan, C. (1982). *In a Different Voice: Psychological Theory and Woman's Development.* Cambridge, MA: Harvard University Press.
Gould, R. (1978). *Transformations, Growth and Change in Adult Life.* New York: Simon & Schuster.

Guntrip, H. (1969). *Schizoid Phenomena, Object-Relations and the Self.* New York: International Universities Press.

Handelman, S. (1980). Intimate distance: the boundary of life and art in "To the Lighthouse." *International Review of Psycho-Analysis* 7:41-49.

Hollander, M. (1970). The need or wish to be held. *Archives of General Psychiatry* 22:445-453.

Horwitz, L. (1990). Psychotherapy as a trial for psychoanalysis. *Psychoanalytic Inquiry* 10:43-66.

Jacobs, T. (1986). On countertransference enactments. *Journal of the American Psychoanalytic Association* 34:289-307.

────── (1991). *The Use of the Self.* Madison, CT: International Universities Press.

Kegan, R. (1982). *The Evolving Self: Problem and Process in Human Development.* Cambridge, MA: Harvard University Press.

Kernberg, O. (1976). Barriers to falling and remaining in love. In *Object Relations Theory and Clinical Psychoanalysis,* pp. 185-213. Northvale, NJ: Jason Aronson.

Lax, E. (1991). Woody and Mia: A New York story. *New York Times Magazine,* 24 February 1991.

Levine, H. (1985). Psychotherapy as the initial phase of a psychoanalysis. *International Review of Psycho-Analysis* 12:285-297.

Loewald, H. (1960). On the therapeutic action of psychoanalysis. *International Journal of Psycho-Analysis* 41:16-33.

Loewenstein, R. (1951). The problem of interpretation. *Psychoanalytic Quarterly* 20:1-14.

Mahler, M. S. (1971). A study of the separation-individuation process and its possible application to borderline phenomenon in the psychoanalytic situation. In *The Selected Papers of Margaret S. Mahler,* vol. 2, pp. 169-187. New York: Jason Aronson.

────── (1972). Rapprochement subphase of the separation-individuation process. In *The Selected Papers of Margaret S. Mahler,* vol. 2, pp. 130-148. New York: Jason Aronson.

────── (1974). Symbiosis and individuation: the psychological birth of the human infant. In *The Selected Papers of Margaret S. Mahler,* vol. 2, pp. 149-165. New York: Jason Aronson.

Mahler, M. S., Pine, F., and Bergman, A. (1975). *The Psychological Birth of the Human Infant.* New York: Basic Books.

Prown, J. (1987). Winslow Homer in his art. *Smithsonian Studies in American Art* 1:30-45.

Pruett, K. (1990). *The impact of involved fatherhood on child development: research and clinical perspectives.* Paper presented at the meeting of the Philadelphia Psychoanalytic Society, October.

Schwaber, E. (1981). Empathy: a mode of analytic listening. *Psychoanalytic Inquiry* 1:357-392.

Stewart, H. (1989). Technique at the basic fault/regression. *International Journal of Psycho-Analysis* 70:221-230.

Tyler, A. (1974). *Celestial Navigation.* New York: Knopf.

────── (1985). *Accidental Tourist.* New York: Knopf.

Waelder, R. (1930). The principle of multiple function: observations on multiple determination. *Psychoanalytic Quarterly* 5:45-62.

Winnicott, D. W. (1960). String: a technique of communication. In *The Maturational Processes and the Facilitating Environment,* pp. 153-157. New York: International Universities Press.

Woolf, V. (1927). *To the Lighthouse.* New York: Harcourt, Brace & World.

4

A PROBLEM WITH THE COUCH: INCAPACITIES AND CONFLICTS

Alvin Frank, M.D.

In this chapter I illustrate the developmental line of an iatrogenic symptom in a particular young woman's analysis. This at first may seem a contradiction in terms. "Developmental line" implies ontogenesis, evolution: "iatrogenic," a topical, situation-related phenomenon, as "induced inadvertently by a physician or his treatment," according to Webster's. I hope to resolve this apparent discrepancy in an effort to bring about an enhanced understanding of both dimensions.

The symptom, which consisted of an inability to lie on the couch, appeared in the beginning and then intermittently during the patient's treatment. At first it occurred regularly, then occasionally. In this review of the case, I have selected those aspects that so vividly illustrate the drama of the child and her most important person, as well as the issues of internalization, separation, and reunion, which are the province of separation–individuation theory. But these constellations impacted unmistakably on later issues, particularly on gender identity, as they were experienced in the phallic and oedipal phases. The odyssey of this particular patient's analysis is the subject of this chapter.

EARLIER OBSERVATIONS

I cannot offer you much in the way of guidelines, for purposes of comparison or contrast, from the published experiences of other analysts. This is somewhat surprising, considering the frequency with which one hears informally of such occurrences. In most indexed references the analyst's couch is used to mean psychoanalysis itself. In contrast, there is an extensive body of writing regarding the other basic technical precept, that of the "fundamental rule" of free association.

Interestingly, Freud's (1913) first recommendation of the couch cited resistance to the procedure: "The patient usually regards being made to adopt this position as a hardship and rebels against it" (p. 134). Most subsequent published reports concern themselves with problems involving the meaning of the couch to the patient. For example, Spitz (1956) proposed that with the couch and free association Freud "created a surprising parallel to the infantile situation," the patient "speaking into the emptiness of space" as does the infant. Not infrequently patients reported to him the feeling of "being humiliatingly *forced* to be a child, . . . and of the feeling that the analyst is a grown-up, . . . sitting up on a higher level, the level of the parent" (p. 382).

Fenichel (1941) advocated treating resistance to lying on the coach as one would a phobia, insisting on talking about it without requiring actual compliance. Glover (1955) suggested that patients sometimes react manifestly to the analytic setting as if a feature were a symbol of a danger situation. He noted that in most instances failures to lie down were minor problems, easily overcome. But more serious instances are those where the reaction has phobic, obsessional, paranoid, or schizoid intensity, or in patients with strong defenses against hetero- or homosexual passive seduction fantasies. Glover's formulations are stated without clinical data, and it is impossible to know what experiences led to them.

Montagnier (1989) described a patient who requested a face-to-face analysis and also occasionally wanted to express himself through drawing rather than orally. He advocated the occasional necessity for such flexibility in order to maintain conditions sustaining "narcissistic and objectal transference." As best as I could tell, use of the couch in this case meant doing it the analyst's way; sitting and drawing represented the patient's self-assertion. Greenson (1965) wrote of a young man who, reacting to the analyst's admission of anger, sat up with his consent. The patient needed several weeks of visual contact to assure himself that the analyst was unlike his father, who had repeatedly assaulted him with a rectal thermometer throughout his childhood. It was also necessary for that analysand to ascertain that the analyst was not sexually excited, angry, or contemptuous as he associated. A patient of Orens (1965) refused to lie on the couch for the first three months or so of analysis. When she did try, she became panicky within a few minutes and sat up. Eventually her difficulty was explained by her presentation of the situation, with the analyst above and behind her, as connoting her helplessness and powerlessness. The involved underlying issues included the patient's inner and projected sadistic impulses, particularly as she fantasized herself castrated and castrating.

McAloon (1987) contributed a detailed account emphasizing her countertransference responses to a patient's refusal over three and a half years to use the couch. The analyst was alternately provoked, frustrated, angry, and guilt-ridden, and experienced profound doubts regarding her own competence and professional identity. The couch issue was only an aspect of the patient's questionable analytic suitability. McAloon was inexperienced, and she was perhaps not as sensitive to the transference issues as to her own. The patient's difficulty in cooperating probably began as a fear of losing control over the analyst. This, and the profound passivity the patient experienced, meant a repetition of his experience with a provocative, genitally exhibitionistic mother. The issue of the couch soon became part of the transference–countertransference interplay, involving particularly sadomasochistic provocations and responses from both parties.

Three examples in the literature focused on a lack of developmental capacities necessary to sustain one's self with the regressions implicit in lying on the couch, particularly without the sustaining view of the analyst. In an article addressed to altered states of consciousness during analysis, Silber (1970) recounted the incident of a patient who, with the failure of defenses, had to rise from the couch and sit in a chair. This enabled him to evaluate reality more effectively and to ward off further regression. In other reported instances the difficulties in using the couch signaled a developmental deficit equivalent to a lack of "the capacity to be alone" in Winnicott's sense (1958). Reiser (1986) wrote of a woman who in four months of face-to-face contact was animated, friendly, and articulate. With the couch and analysis she became concrete, complaining, and passively resistant. These were the manifestations of a defensive altered ego state dating from childhood. The loss of visual contact with the analyst impacted on the vulnerabilities and memories resulting from growing up with an abusive father and repeated experiences of separation, physical confinement, and overstimulation. After a year and a half of therapy the analyst suggested returning to the psychotherapeutic mode, and the patient was able to again work comfortably and effectively.

In the third example, Weissman (1977) described a patient whose need for visual contact shaped her analysis. He attributed this reaction to the patient's three-month separation from her mother before her first birthday and the experience of growing up with two depressed parents. Neither patient nor analyst anticipated, after four anamnestic diagnostic interviews, that "all hell would break loose when [the patient] lay down and lost facial contact" with the analyst (p. 428). At first the patient took a blanket from the foot of the couch and covered herself, yielding it only reluctantly after promising never to do it again. Her posture was a picture of discomfort and tension, and the sessions were filled with anxiety and depressive anguish as she experienced loss and isolation without the analyst in sight. The patient sat up for two periods at her initiative, with the analyst employing a careful interpretive neutrality. The first period, of three months' duration, followed the analyst's vacation at the end of the first analytic year. It was preceded by the observation during the ninth month of the patient's "hungry need" for facial contact. The patient decided to return to the couch with the emergence of profound concern over loss of self and strong sexual feelings and fantasies during the sessions. The second period covered the fourth and fifth years of analysis. The decision to use the couch was presented by the patient as representing a new assertiveness, yet on a few occasions when she agreed to use the couch she responded masochistically and was unable to work. This constellation was recognizable as signifying hateful compliance with the analyst's implied demand. At this point, of course, the couch had taken on a separate meaning. The patient terminated analysis successfully, with recognition of the meaning of termination as a repetition of childhood loss.

CLINICAL PRESENTATION[1]

As in Weissman's account, I had no premonition in the instance I present here that lying on the couch would involve more than eventless cooperation with a conventional, technically indicated practice. The analysand in this case history sought help because of chronic intermittent anxiety and depression, which had been

---

1. The material is derived from notes dictated immediately after each session. The extent of note taking varied from hour to hour, depending on the amount of time available to the analyst. Notes range from a half to two single-spaced pages. The analysis occurred four times a week and followed usual technical procedures. There is no fictionalizing or alteration of data in this account.

A Problem with the Couch

troublesome since adolescence. Having explained this, to quote my notes at the time,

> she quickly interposes that this is the result of her outrageous parents' outrageous behavior—specifically her father, who is a "bastard." The father is a professional man, and according to the patient she has wanted help since her teen years but the father has manipulated her in such a way that she didn't get [the help]. . . . The mother is described as a masochist, beaten down by the father's cruelty. She spent little time with the patient during her childhood, worked for a number of years, and then went into [her occupation]. The father is interested only in [his profession] and social position: the parents are generous only with money. On the other hand, [the patient] says, her parents use money to maintain control over her life.
>
> A couple . . . joined the family household when the patient was 6 months old. She feels very close to both of them: they are two of the three people in the world to whom she can openly express her feelings. [The third is her husband.] There was a constant emphasis during her childhood on not expressing or showing feelings, in consequence of which the patient made an agreement with herself that she'd never tell anyone about her real feelings.

The patient was also afraid of repeating her parents' mistakes should she have children. She mentioned two brothers, born when she 3 and 7. Both siblings were sickly as infants and children, the youngest seriously so.

> While always active socially, the patient had managed to maintain "a very platonic level" with men until meeting her husband, whom she had married a year before analysis. She was very concerned about the impact of her problems on him. I learned in subsequent sessions that although he was only slightly younger than her, he had not achieved her career status and was financially and emotionally dependent. In our first session she described scapegoating him with angry attacks. Within a few

weeks I learned that this included striking him. When he became angry with her, she reacted as to a personal rejection. On those occasions she retreated into days of solitude and silent animosity. Despite these problems she described herself as sexually satisfied.

I noted the patient's focus on the father's mistreatment and her obvious pleasure as she "gleefully" detailed "many incidents [in which] the father was cruel and [physically] hurt her...." "This young woman ... has already formulated her case on the basis of her mistreatment by her parents," my summary states. Her formulation was a historical psychologically dictated compromise formation, equivalent to what Kris (1956) called a personal myth.

There was a four-month gap between the two anamnestic sessions and the start of analysis, the result of the patient's request for time to arrange schedules, finances, and her vacation. In the second session I had explained to her the use of the couch and free association. She expressed concern at the time about free association but did not mention the couch. She said that she was afraid of expressing her feelings spontaneously, particularly of her inner aggression. She also was concerned about whether she could perform adequately.

The patient began the first session by leaving the door of the office open, asking if she should close it, laughing, closing the door, looking at the couch, and wondering whether or not she should lie on it. I sat down and acknowledged that she was concerned about lying on the couch. She laughed, then said she had a problem lying down which she hadn't mentioned, then laughed again. She said she often needed encouragement and asked me for directions. I said that I recognized she was anxious, had a problem in lying down, and wanted to put the decision in my hands. She sat down on a chair, told at some length about a summer visit home, wondered if she should tell her superiors about analysis, and asked me again what to do. I said that I knew that she was anxious about getting started and wanted me to structure the situation. She walked to the couch, sat on it, spoke of her anxiety, asked if she should take off her shoes, and responded to my conjecture that she was testing me by then lying down. She spoke of her concern about getting away with things with people, asked a number of questions, and talked about needing the company of radio and TV when alone at home. She said she did not know me well enough to be sure that she could trust me. With people she trusted she could remain silent. She then sat halfway up and said she would do so unless I told her not to. I recognized her anxiety, which resulted in her need to continue to test the situation. Then she spoke of her loneliness, how unhappy she was, how she had so few friends, and wondered if people liked her. I applied this to her concern about being liked by and liking me. She seemed startled and denied either was of importance. As we agreed that we were touching on feelings that she feared and generally avoided, she gradually lay down on the couch. At the end of the session she said she was glad it was over, yet she felt she had wasted precious time.

I was thrown somewhat off balance by this experience, feeling in a way that whatever I did or didn't do might misfire. The patient was obviously frightened and wanted my support in the form of requesting demands for performance and controls to alleviate her anxiety. She also seemed to desperately need the contact with me for its own value, whatever that might be. I wondered whether she might actually fear being lonely on the couch without me in sight. At the same time, I was aware of her need to provoke me and replicate the relationship reported with her father. I believed that her problem with the couch could condense important dynamic constellations as suggested by her first remarks. Either excusing her or forcing her to comply with the practice would be suppressive and probably work against analysis.

Over the next weeks and months my understanding was largely confirmed, and I was generally able to do more than simply avoid countertransference errors. I soon learned that the patient's problem with the couch could not be artificially isolated from other transferential material and required analysis in relation to the whole picture. Considering the distortions inherent in any presentation's focus on a particular symptom, I ask the reader to apply the material quoted in the broader implied contexts.

In these first days of analysis the patient observed that she understood her wish to get questions and answers from me as a way to avoid silence. Her problem in lying down at home at night was actually a problem in falling asleep. First, she had to cover herself from head to toe to control her anxiety. She slept poorly at night, better during the day.

At some sessions during this period she never lay on the couch. Usually, though, she was up and down. She also continued to cite her fear of her feelings. By the tenth session she was aware of confusing me with her father and spontaneously spoke of her unwillingness to lie on the couch as a continuation of her struggles with him. To lie down, then, could mean surrender and humiliation. But she also volunteered that often if people were out of her sight it was as if they did not exist. After our third weekend interval she said that it was as if she had to get to know me all over again; I was somehow different. Her immediate associations were to her intolerance of her father.

After missing a session because of illness, she began by "fixing" my image as she lay down on the couch to be sure that I was there, that it was safe. She ended this hour before a weekend by visualizing a pet dog who had died when she was 7 years old lying dead on the floor. The patient could not lie down the following Monday session, described a "horrible" weekend, and blamed it on her humiliating "dependency" on me; I had moved too close to her. Now she told me the first dream of the analysis: "My fish was dying—it's an angel fish—I love it, I take wonderful care of it, it was dying, lying on its side and going down. I told my husband to do something about it and he wouldn't do anything."

The patient spontaneously associated to her anger and anxiety with her husband and co-workers, and I suggested that she was displacing these feelings from me. She paused, agreed, and told me a dream from Friday or Saturday night: "I remember it hazily—I was somewhere—I wanted to get back to someplace—I didn't want to miss anything."

She paused, smiled, and said she had just remembered saying the previous week that she did not want to miss appointments here. (Clearly, loss meant death to the patient, and death meant lying down.) She continued with another dream of separation and reunion.

This discussion was largely forgotten at the next session. The patient was afraid she might fall asleep on the couch, and recalled a pubertal boyfriend toward whom she could not express feelings.

Her ambivalence continued to be expressed over the next few months. No weekend went unnoticed. One could be deliriously happy, as she anticipated our reunion, or furious and abysmal, as she felt my absence. She pictured me as impatient and angry, shoving her down on the couch, or as handsome, warm, practical, and pleasurable. Her admissions of envy, cruelty, and bitchiness with her husband and brothers evolved into a wish to be "mean" to me. She said she was frustrated by not hearing my groans as she turned the screws. That was the type of child she now remembered herself as having been: vile, sarcastic, mocking, and angry. A dream including the word "rejection" led to picturing rejected children and then, with sadness, to picturing herself as a rejected child. She did not remember feeling that way at the time; she had believed it was only much later, in her teen years.

Over time she revealed more about her concern with lying down to sleep. She spoke about childhood nightmares. Her mother would awaken her during these dreams, and she now had difficulty going to sleep without her husband present. Her next association was of biting her nails as a child.

In these months, the patient demonstrated a number of incapacities manifested as her problem in lying down. In the most extreme form, if I was out of sight I might be out of mind and terrifyingly lost; my psychological image could change with loss of my visual image. This problem was repeatedly linked to her anger and intensely ambivalent needs. My voice was solicited through request and provocation; like the comforting presence of radio and TV, it could ease her fearful state of aloneness. Her sleep symptom involved the fear of giving up the external world and objects, also represented as death, through not having her mother or her substitutes.

The disturbances of object constancy could thus be so profound as to undermine their neuropsychological underpinnings, those equivalent to Piaget's (1936) "object permanence."[2] Mahler and colleagues (1975) described a 2-year-old girl for whom the same was true: ". . . it seemed that momentarily she not only lacked emotional object constancy, but also that she lost its cognitive counterpart, Piaget's 'mental image of the absent object'" (p. 162). The changes reported in my visual image, paralleling those of my personal image, were reminiscent of Anna Freud's (Arlow et al. 1968) cautionary anecdote about maintaining object constancy despite stress. Freud told of how, during a discussion with children of why they kept family photographs on their mantelpieces, a 4- or 5-year-old girl, separated from her parents, volunteered: "That is so that you don't think they have gone all nasty when you haven't seen them for a long time" (p. 507).

The object constancy, which is a usual acquisition of the third year and the condition for progression from rapprochement, requires much more than this neuropsychological prerequisite, the capacity to retain the absent love object's visual representation. "It . . . implies the unifying of the 'good' and 'bad' object into one whole representation" (Mahler et al. 1975, p. 110), that is, the tempering of infantile hateful and destructive drives. Repeatedly, the analysand's associations, dreams, and actions, as well as the fluctuations of the transference, demonstrated a lack of this capacity.

The weekends in particular played out the passions of the problematic rapprochement phase, externally imposed by analytic scheduling. The internally motivated equivalent was de-

---

2. I had earlier experience (see Frank 1987) with the analysis of another young woman with failed developmental capacity for object constancy, heralded by problems in remembering faces. In that instance it was due to prosopagnosia, a rare neurologic deficit consisting of an inability to recognize or evoke the facial images of the most familiar persons in one's life. I wondered at the time if lightning could strike twice, but that was not the case.

monstrable in the patient's alternating self-contempt and resulting self-assertions over what she feared was passivity and neediness, and angry provocative demand for the satisfactions they represented. But when she was absent on her own initiative, which was more than occasional, she did not miss me. To the contrary, whatever the reason and however arbitrary, such absences were presented as the unchallengeable exercise of her autonomy, and not uncommonly as challenges to hold on to her.

More meanings began to emerge. Noting that she cried now over hurts, she fantasized about my triumphant pleasure. To cry was to be feminine, weak, exploited, and ignored like her mother. As a child she remembered feeling more like a boy than a girl. A dream began: "There was something wrong with my eyes, they needed an operation. . . ." Her first association was to her mother's eye being torn by a thorn and not being given proper care by her father. A few minutes later it became obvious from her associations that she was sitting up in the dream. I asked her about this, and she said that was odd, because one should be lying down for a procedure like that. She burst out laughing as she observed that the eye operation must refer to the analysis. Yet she also identified with and projected the image of her mother as a phallic harpy. The same dream concluded: "Three women were operating on [her mother's eyes]. They had a big, big syringe—about 1 inch wide and 4 inches long."

The patient said she felt that I disciplined her by not talking but in the process gave her so much rope that she would hang herself. Was I very impatient with her for not lying down? She predicted that when she did so it would be because of her fear of my impatience, to satisfy me, rather than for her own benefit.

She clearly perceived me as the pregenital mother, replete with problems in identification, shamefulness, and rivalry for her nurturing satisfactions. There had been projection of the analysand's punitiveness, withholding, sadism, and rejection onto me as this person. With interpretation a much more respectable, likable, giving mother emerged. Despite her anger the patient reported awakening and crying out for her mother, and was embarrassed. Her mother's generosity to one of her brothers led to intense anger and jealousy; she hated *his* greediness and insatiability. Legends of his harassments were replaced by memories of her physical attacks on both siblings.

A sequence was soon observable. The patient regularly turned in the transference from her mother for nurturance to her father. This was then quickly complicated by the conflicts of sexual curiosity, desire, and prohibition. Similarly, rivalry with her siblings was very often conflated with oedipal competition. For example, in the fifth month of analysis she told of the following dream:

My father and brother [were] at the dinner table. [My brother] asked my father, "Why don't you like me?" My father said, "You've always been a thorn in the sole of my foot." [My brother] was hurt a lot. . . . It was a cruel thing to say. My father never liked him.

And yet another dream:

It had to do with my mother's first engagement ring. My mother gave it to [that same brother]. I was absolutely furious. . . . I as the oldest and the daughter and should be getting it.

Now the patient began reacting to me more consistently as her recalled father of childhood, a transference that by and large persisted through the remainder of the analysis. She permitted herself a forbidden anxious curiosity about me and dreaded she might be getting possessive. At the same time, her possessiveness toward her husband took the form of fear of his sexual infidelity and loss. She recalled childhood dreams that added a phobic sexual dimension to her problems of lying down and sleeping in bed. I had a bunk bed. I had repetitive dreams that the bed was hurled out of a hayloft by someone, falling, falling, falling, until I woke up just before hitting the ground. I had other dreams of a snake under my bed, wanting to crawl under the covers. She then thought of a time of waiting for her father at twilight. After a minute's silence she mentioned marijuana. Just before smoking it she always had a feeling that it was a forbidden thing. During her next session she asked me to do what she presented as a forbidden thing, to write her a prescription. In fact, she had earlier confessed her fear that I would connect not lying on the couch with "some sexual thing." She anticipated that any discussion of sex could lead to my calling her frigid or, paradoxically, an obsessed nymphomaniac.

The patient feared her deepening attachment to me. She recalled how her mother recently ridiculed her when she embraced and kissed her father. She dreamed that night that I asked her to bring some money. Money, she interjected, was used in her family to show affection. I interpreted this as her wish to show me affection, and her thoughts turned to her hostility toward her mother.

Lying on the couch now carried the meaning of sexual surrender. She was a "slut" because men found her attractive, and reported that women complained because her skirt was short and men turned on to her. During one session she lay awkwardly on the couch, leaning on her arm. She had wanted to put her head on the pillow from the beginning but felt that it would be like succumbing sexually to me. A few months later she did not lie down because of her conscious fear the it would be pleasurable, and once experienced could never be resisted.

Soon issues of gender were more and more complicated by the relationship with her father as reexperienced in the transference. This involved not only the themes but their intensity. She believed her body, like her mother's—particularly her breasts and genitals—was ugly and flabby. Women's bodies could be beautiful only from the back. Her menstrual fluid was represented by a dead fish, smelly and horrible. Later her vagina was represented in a dream by a puncture wound, blue and ugly, which she knew would bleed again; then she would bleed to death. In her dreams she repeatedly asserted manifestly or symbolically that she had a penis. Her clear unconscious wish was to be my little boy. In dreams referring to the analysis in the second year she pictured herself as a crippled man, as a paraplegic needing patience, and as herself being fitted for a pants suit by an incompetent seamstress. She hatefully believed men to be better than women, and envied what she asserted was my superior intelligence.

During this period she spoke of an "incestuous family," whose father forced his daughters to lie in bed with him until they were 14 years old. One feared pregnancy because of a fantasy of sexual interaction with him. The patient was furious the next session and sat up throughout, accusing me of misbehaving with her associations. From this time there was ongoing recollection of her childhood sexual exhibitionism, curiosity, and misdemeanors. She now wanted to sit up because looking at me was gratifying. Within a month there were recollections of looking at her father's genitals during childhood, of perhaps showering with him when she was very young, and of stealing looks while he slept nude. Reviewing the material was like rereading Galenson and Roiphe's (1980) developmental observations on the pre-oedipal genital phase of the boy in rapprochement.

This struggle shaped the presentation of both negative and positive oedipal strivings. When the patient learned of an acquaintance, a woman, contacting me for an appointment toward the end of the first year of analysis, she was distraught with jealousy and rage. The next week she "couldn't" lie down at first. She had a manifest dream of disparaging men as disappointing and of making love to this woman with something "just as good" as what a man had, her own penis. In one felt swoop she had solved everything: she had me by excluding me from the triangle, had won the woman, had acquired a penis, and had fantasied satisfactions at every level.

She also dreamed of hard penises that excited her as a woman, manifestly her father's and mine, early into the second year. She spoke of a passionate wish that I attack and "mutilate" her. She wanted to lie back and do nothing, and wanted me to do "everything." Then she could sleep—she wanted to omit her next association—as after orgasm. She stated that she could not tolerate feeling so passive and sat up. In her life outside analysis she permitted herself to be demeaned regularly and humiliated sexually. Six months later she stated that her modesty concealed her wish to attract me. She felt intensely ashamed, and within a few minutes talked about her body as shameful and ugly. As she continued to feel competition with other women for me, longstanding self-defeating attitudes, often rationalized by a narcissistic assertment that she would not compete unless assured of victory, were articulated.

In addition to guilt, to want me sexually was ferociously complicated by pregenital hungers. Wanting to displace and destroy other women reinvoked the condensed issue of her frustrated need-laden rage toward her own mother and its shameful and guilty complications. Pregnancy wishes and fantasies were complicated by rage over her mother's having given birth. To an extraordinary degree pregenital hatred and narcissism were confused with oedipal; the common expressive modalities were those of oral and anal sadism, defiance, and withholding experienced internally or projectively. This was particularly noteworthy in the context of Mahler and colleagues' (1975) rapprochement subphase with attendant issues of dependent adhesion versus autonomy. Absolutely characteristic were the pronounced separation reactions; the patient's anxious need to watch me, termed "shadowing" when observed in these toddlers; the alternation of fierce wishes for reunion and equally powerful fears of engulfment; the provocative "darting away," as well as exaggerated and anal aggression and negativism. It included, of course, being played out in her sitting or lying.

An important example of such overdetermination was the patient's original psychological organization of orgasm. She believed herself a "slut" with her husband when she responded to his desires, and was anorgasmic. This meant she wanted a man and had successfully competed for him by arousing his passion. On one such occasion she suddenly felt as if she were being raped and began screaming and yelling. She was now the victim, not the guilty victimizer. However, when sex was at her initiative, and for her alone, she knew she would be orgasmic. Then she would relax her controls; it would be a predictable, pleasurable experience. She had redesigned a guilt-filled, competitive oedipal experience, first as dyadic and masochistic, then as if she were having a bowel movement on her initiative alone while ignoring and withholding from the man. Her experienced autonomy in the form of defiant self-determination was the condition of the very pregenital narcissistic fulfillment she simultaneously disavowed.

As time went on we were able to piece together her "real" story, a reconstruction that explained her psychopathology as presented as analytic experience. Her father had indeed been the center of her emotional life, as she had originally described. But his important impact was in a warm, even adoring, caring mode rather than as a "bastard." In part this had compensated for the loss of attention from her mother in her first two years because of a chronic infectious disease diagnosed during the patient's infancy. The illness had mandated the mother's hospitalization and prolonged invalidism. The mother's recovery was accompanied by the birth of a son, a sickly infant who received most of her time and attention. The couple referred to had been present and invaluable and loved caretakers who actually arrived on the scene when the patient was in the last half of her second year. But the center of the patient's universe until something happened in the first part of latency was her father. We came to understand that problems of identification and sexual identity were thus confused in her mind.

The family, as you have read, had included an aggressive, sometimes abusive, controlling presence. It was the patient herself, as she remembered, and substantiated by others' accounts and even home movies viewed "by chance." What had happened? The patient's earlier experiences had sensitized her to all issues of separation, loss, and competition as forcefully complicating autonomous assertion. This was compounded by confusing and conflicted issues of identity complicated by those of gender. If she could continue to be her admired father's favored older "son," she both had him and was like him. However, she was now faced with the birth of still another boy, one who immediately became the source of very anxious preoccupation from both of her parents. It concurrently led to an angry reaction because of the disappointment of the young girl's oedipal strivings, another loss of a different meaning, conflated with, and epitomized by, this evidence of her parents' intimacy. Clearly, the original accounts of her father's mistreatments included thinly disguised masochistic sexual fantasies. These "many incidents where the father was cruel and (physically) hurt her" were not recounted after the first telling. They were obvious projections and masochistic embellishments played out by a provocative child who sometimes did arouse her father's ire.

The family-imposed restraint on expressing feelings turned out to be largely fabrication, the rationalized motive for another area of the patient's willful withholding. It was operative in the sexual stinginess that explained her "very platonic" teasing of men. Furthermore, her selection of a husband had very purposefully mandated exactly what she got: an immature, vulnerable man with whom she could reenact the aggression, hatred, and guilt originally felt toward her younger brothers, as well as those displaced from her parents. The best she could do was to settle for the lowest common denominator—the limitations, passions, and hatreds of the very young child whose screams could be felt and heard in the adult analysand's sessions.

The overdetermined symptom represented as her problem with the couch had both aspects of structural deficit related to developmental incapacities and classical compromise formations based on the meaning of the experience. Structural regressions were in consequence of an ego already compromised by developmental fixations and incapacities currently impacted by powerful affects. Without the analyst in sight she experienced the object world as lost; she could not depend on it to provide the illusion of structuring lent by external reality. It was as if she were home alone in the dark, uncovered, not hearing the radio, not seeing the television. She was like the children described by Fraiberg (1950), unable to sleep because of the paucity of structure that predisposes to the "traumatic situation ... that of helplessness, the experience of being overwhelmed and indefensible" (p. 287). Mahler and La Perriere (1965) viewed this disturbance as indicative "of the child's progressive individuation and of his defense against the threat of symbiotic fusion represented by sleep," and as specific to rapprochement (p. 488).

The succession of meaning-laden compromise formations described above, representing drives and conflicts up and down the psychosexual and genetic scales, continued to convey the impact of this less-developed period in two other important ways. One was in the intensity, the ferocity, the economic aspects of the patient's presentations. The other was the confusion of themes, the too facile and ready movement between constellations that was so much a feature of the first half of analysis. The psyche's very organization was stamped with the impressions of the mind's first years. Until analyzed and worked through, the crying baby and young child were always lurking in the background, shaping each expression and experience.

> The problem with the couch was gradually resolved, as were other areas of symptomatology, as analysis continued. Then suddenly, in the last part of the fourth analytic year, "all hell broke loose" again, although not with the original intensity. In particular the patient was angry and defiant, asserting that I made no difference at all to her and did not care about her anyway. Only after months of confusion did we come up with the precipitant: she had begun to plan on termination. She did then consider the issue over the next three weeks and decided to stop in about five months. Now, with a fraction of the work originally expended, symptoms were again replaced by the thoughts and feelings they represented. A special case was that of the organizing theme of termination. My willingness to let her go, and her anticipation of my absence, signified rejection at each developmental level. She was that discarded, forgotten baby, toddler, little boy and girl, schoolchild, teenager, and adult. She enviously and resentfully speculated about who would replace her.
>
> She began the last session, lying on the couch, saying that she wanted to keep it superficial and intellectual and avoid her feelings about leaving. A reaction must come, but only later. She then began to cry, as she had cried in many recent sessions, and

continued crying as she talked about experiencing termination as my death. I cited her anger toward me for letting her go, as well as her fear of losing me. I observed that she was determined that no one should have me after her. I understood she would feel my loss as a death. Now her anger and sadness about leaving were expressed with her gratitude and feeling of accomplishment. Her tears could no longer be said to lie too deep for words as she lay on the couch this last time.

The patient had a sustaining prediction through the termination phase. In a city like ours, really a big small town, our paths would surely cross, she felt. In fact, well over a decade has passed without our meeting. I heard indirectly about five or six years later that she looked well, and spoke animatedly and with pleasure of the challenges and satisfactions of her new life.

COMMENTS

This case is an exception to the conventional expectation that significant inability to collaborate in usual analytic procedure is a profoundly negative prognostic indicator. But the experience is not inconsistent with the limited number of more or less detailed case studies that were summarized earlier. Even if one excludes Greenson's and Silber's cases as representing time-limited circumscribed episodes in analyses well under way, the odds still seem to favor productive analysis in such situations. This could be a reflection, however, of reporting biased toward publication of positive results, if only because such patients remain in treatment long enough, and give enough information, so that a report is instructive.

While previous accounts emphasize either impaired ego capacities or classic compromise formations of meaningful dynamic content, this case provided material that substantiated both elements. Furthermore, while other cases in general cite a particular internal constellation within, or without, a corresponding period or circumstance, this analysis demonstrated what could be compared to a developmental line in the genesis of the patient's problem with the couch.

This observation introduces the issue of the choice of symptom, an area where we too often must fall back on unprovable citations of endowment. That element was certainly present here: the patient's high energy level, adaptability, intelligence, and creativity as demonstrated by her ability to utilize the analytic process. Of particular note was her use of the rapprochement phase as a template in the shaping and organizing of her emotional life as initially described and played out in the analysis. The patient came to this developmental phase so compromised and vulnerable that transit was bound to be difficult. Her vulnerability involved the ego impairments resulting from the fierce needs and antagonisms provoked through the inconstancy of her nurturers, as well as those drives' continuing power. Her most important caring person was her father, with whom interactions were limited too much to evenings and weekends. The identifications with him were her most important. Her gender identity was confused and ambivalent; she navigated the rapprochement pre-oedipal genital phase more as a boy than as a girl. Add to this the patient's felt shamefulness of her longings and their equation with her immobilized mother, who *could not* do other than lie in bed, as she herself years later *would not* lie on the couch.

Contemporaneous with rapprochement, her refound mother's recovery was associated with a brother's birth; now object loss and hunger were fueled by still more frustration, hatred, and envy. Further confusion was introduced by two new caretakers. Consider then the problematic status of object constancy, an internal achievement normatively providing progression from rapprochement and phasic reorganization.

The patient greeted the phallic and oedipal stages with an augmented intensity; an unsure and conflict-laden sense of gender: a pregenital confusion of needs, alms, and motives: and an entrenched narcissistic and dyadic object fixation. Both the positive and negative Oedipus complexes were complicated by her unresolved masculine entrenchment and pregenital aggression toward both parents; the oedipal triadic competition was too much experienced as rivalries with a sibling, or as power struggles of the anal and oral stages, or as extraordinary narcissistic assertion and vulnerability. The primitive qualities of the parental representations were internalized in the form of a savagely punitive superego. And all of the foregoing was largely initially acted in and out and experienced and represented in the idiom of rapprochement as an organizing frame of reference.

Those of our colleagues who have provided developmental observations, schema, and propositions have given psychoanalysis an extraordinary and invaluable tool for application in the analytic situation. Freud's knowledge of infants and children was largely limited to prevalent nineteenth-century pediatrics, subservient to the culture and times. Only occasionally could he draw on direct observations of children, such as his own grandchild, or on supervision of others directly involved with children, as the junior colleague whose son had a fear of horses. Analytically informed studies of infants and children, as exemplified by those based on separation–individuation theory, bestow upon contemporary analysis a corpus of learning garnered from the vantage point of careful, systematic observations. As the result of our colleagues' efforts, we are better able to fill in the gaps and to understand, treat, and prevent illness. This report is an example. We are in their debt.

REFERENCES

Arlow, J. A., Freud, A., Lampl-de-Groot, J., et al. (1968). Panel discussion. *International Journal of Psycho-Analysis* 49:506–512.

Fenichel, O. (1941). *Problems of Psychoanalytic Technique.* New York: Psychoanalytic Quarterly.

Fraiberg, S. (1950). On the sleep disturbances of early childhood. *Psychoanalytic Study of the Child* 5:285–309. New York: International Universities Press.

Frank, A. (1987). Facial image and object constancy: a clinical experience and a developmental inference. *Psychoanalytic Quarterly* 56:477–496.

Freud, S. (1913). On beginning the treatment (further recommendations on the technique of psycho-analysis). *Standard Edition* 12:121–144.

Galenson, E., and Roiphe, H. (1980). The pre-oedipal development of the boy. *Journal of the American Psychoanalytic Association* 28:805–827.

Glover, E. (1955). *The Technique of Psychoanalysis.* New York: International Universities Press.

Greenson, R. (1965). The working alliance and the transference neurosis. *Psychoanalytic Quarterly* 34:155–181.

Kris, E. (1956). The personal myth: a problem in psychoanalytic technique. *Journal of the American Psychoanalytic Association* 4:653–681.

Mahler, M., and La Perriere, K. (1965). Mother–child interaction during separation-individuation. *Psychoanalytic Quarterly* 34:483–498.

Mahler, M., Pine, F., and Bergman, A. (1975). *The Psychological Birth of the Human Infant: Symbiosis and Individuation.* New York: Basic Books.

McAloon, R. (1987). The need to feel like an analyst: a study of countertransference in the case of a patient who refused to use the couch. *Modern Psychoanalysis* 12:65–87.

Montagnier, M. T. (1989). Bateaux. *Revue Française de Psychanalyse* 53:1209–1217.

Orens, M. (1965). Setting a termination date—an impetus to analysis. *Journal of the American Psychoanalytic Association* 3:651–665.

Piaget, J. (1936). *The Origins of Intelligence in Children.* New York: International Universities Press, 1952.

Reiser, L. (1986). "Lying and lying": a case report of a paradoxical reaction to the couch. *Psychoanalytic Study of the Child* 41:537–559. New Haven: Yale University Press.

Silber, A. (1970). Functional phenomenon: historical concept, contemporary defense. *Journal of the American Psychoanalytic Association* 18:519–537.

Spitz, R. (1956). Transference: the analytic setting and its prototype. *International Journal of Psycho-Analysis* 37:380–385.

Weissman, S. (1977). Face to face: the role of vision and the smiling response. *Psychoanalytic Study of the Child* 32:421–450. New Haven: Yale University Press.

Winnicott, D. (1958). The capacity to be alone. *International Journal of Psycho-Analysis* 39:416–420.

5

UNRESOLVED SEPARATION-INDIVIDUATION, MASOCHISM, AND DIFFICULTY WITH COMPLIANCE

Discussion of Frank's Chapter, "A Problem with the Couch: Incapacities and Conflicts"

LeRoy J. Byerly, M.D.

An intricate blending of pre-oedipal and oedipal issues is the hallmark of the case described by Dr. Alvin Frank in Chapter 4. His central theme draws our attention to the fundamental problem of the couch in analysis. One of the interesting aspects of this case is that until Dr. Frank's patient actually began using the couch, it was not suspected that this would be a problem. The patient's initial fears were not, however, of lying down on the couch, but of expressing her feelings and of being inadequate to the task demanded of her by the analytic process. In this sense, the patient demonstrated a more than usual problem with the "fundamental rule" (Freud 1912, p. 115) of analysis.

Dr. Frank points out the paucity of literature on patients who have had difficulty using the couch. He notes that the problem itself is common enough and every analyst has encountered some resistance from his patients in using the couch. Why such encounters are so poorly documented is an open question. Perhaps the very basic and common nature of the problem detracts attention from it. Another reason for meager attention toward this matter might be that difficulty in lying on the couch encroaches upon the broader issue of ubiquitous difficulties in following the fundamental rule when beginning an analysis. In our analytic thinking, free association is the central factor of importance; lying on the couch is a facilitator of free association.[1] As such, the couch is a secondary, supportive feature to the primary rule of free association.

We might argue that an important aspect of technique is raised by such noncompliance. However, such technical issues become subordinated to our concern with the meaning of the noncompliance. Rather than make active intervention, it is safer for us to assume that this noncompliance will take its place in the overall general resistance and to await the development in the analysis. Frequently, the emphasis shifts from the patient's behavior to countertransference problems that can be critical. Indeed, as in Dr. Frank's patient, the inability to lie on the couch became encompassed in the general resistances and conflicts and was played out in the transference. Under certain circumstances, it would appear that the inability to utilize the couch can become a more or less specific resistance, particularly when countertransference problems become critical. Countertransference problems are most often centered on issues of aggression and control. Aggression and control are inherent in the use of the couch in psychoanalysis. That is, submission is built into the couch, with the patient lying down and the analyst sitting. It is also built into the language of psychoanalysis, which from its earliest days describes the patient as "submitting" to analysis. These countertransference problems are compounded when the analyst is less experienced and has problems in trusting the analytic method. Under these circumstances, technical issues

---

1. The couch may act as more than a facilitator of free association. In ways that are less well understood, it may also act to induce transitional phenomena and precipitate altered states of consciousness that more directly stimulate the free association process.

become overdetermined and are quickly drawn into conflict. A second group of individuals who have difficulty dealing with the couch includes those who have early developmental failures, deficiencies, or traumas. Dr. Frank's patient is representative of this group.

THE MEANING OF LYING DOWN

Before we look at Dr. Frank's clinical case, we might consider some of the technical aspects and meanings that lying on the couch has in the analytic situation. Generally, lying on the couch is thought of in terms of its regressive and submissive qualities. In reviewing Freud's reasons for using the couch, some not so apparent aspects of the meaning of lying down are revealed (Roazen 1975, pp. 82, 123). First, the couch was a remnant from Freud's use of hypnosis, since it permitted the patient to relax and free associate without being burdened by face-to-face confrontation. The residual features of hypnosis were linked to free associational methods. Features common to hypnosis, such as boundary shifts, altered states of consciousness, and hypnagogic phenomena, became part of the transference reaction in the new technique. The couch became the transition between these two treatment methods. The aura of mysticism was also carried from hypnosis to analysis by use of the couch.

Second, Freud viewed the couch as ceremonial. For Freud, ritual served a positive function. The repetitious procedure of lying on the couch became part of the reliability and predictability of the analytic process. The ritualistic use of the couch separated the analytic dialogue from everyday face-to-face conversations.

Third, the couch permitted Freud to keep the "optimal distance" (Bouvet 1958) he required to maintain his commitment to neutrality. This distance facilitated what he regarded as rational insights. It is reported that Freud paid little or no attention to gestures and preverbal signs, much preferring the power of words. In his technique, Freud saw the couch as an opportunity to make such verbal demands on his patients. Additionally, this distance allowed Freud to regulate his empathic responses. He maintained that this stance permitted him to work with a wider range of patients.

Freud considered the hardships imposed by free association, including lying on the couch, justifiable, in that, for most patients, free association was an easier way of temporarily suspending reality, and the responsibility of having to deal with reality. Among the multiply determined reasons for some patients' inability to utilize the couch, the fear of losing contact with reality is an important one. As Dr. Frank's patient demonstrates, however, the resistances associated with fear of losing control and fear of losing contact with reality are drawn from every level of development. Such resistances are not only multiply determined but also demonstrate "change of function" (Hartmann 1958, p. 25), serving different purposes at different developmental levels, as is reflected in the transference. One might conclude, in an oversimplified but meaningful manner, that the inability to use the couch is related to a more basic difficulty with the fundamental rule of psychoanalysis.

Finally, the couch, as the touchstone of psychoanalysis, is regarded by many analysts as necessary for an analytic procedure. The free association method and the couch became inseparable. The following quote of Freud's thoughts about the fate of analysis in America contains these same sentiments.

> Freud's forebodings about that would happen to his ideas in America have been in some measure fulfilled. For example, in the consulting rooms in present day of British Analysts, the analytic couch is prominently displayed sometimes in the very center of the room. When one moves across the Atlantic to New England, the analytic couch, still a distinct entity, is more likely to be inconspicuously placed against a wall. In Chicago, an analyst's couch might be used for social purposes as well as therapeutic

ones, and on the West Coast, the furniture of the analyst's office, which is likely to include enough chairs for group therapy, makes abundantly clear just what Freud feared that to the analyst, the practice of analysis has become only one therapy, among many others. [Roazen 1975, p. 388]

A DISORDER OF OBJECT CONSTANCY?

Dr. Frank's case has many interesting and intriguing facets that are difficult to bring together under one single formulation. As Dr. Frank notes, however, that the issues of internalization, separation, and reunion draw our attention to separation–individuation. The resistance in using the couch and other general resistances in the transference point more clearly to problems and failures in the developmental line of individuation. In fact, I would propose that Dr. Frank's patient can be classified as having a disorder of object constancy. It is appropriate here to take note of Mahler's (1977) criteria for libidinal object constancy: (a) self-constancy leads to individual entity and identity; (b) object constancy facilitates triangular, whole object relations; (c) there is a flexible, narcissistic, genital orientation in terms of psychosexual development; and (d) repression as a major defensive mechanism replaces splitting mechanisms. These characteristics features of object constancy are not present in Dr. Frank's patient. Rather, she demonstrates a failure of object constancy in the persistence of ambivalence and ambitendency, the presence of a poor self-image, and marked difficulties in negotiating and establishing self/other boundaries.

Kramer (1980) described a group of adolescent girls with object constancy problems. In this group, the prevalence of splitting, as a pathological defense, interfered with the adolescents' ability to attain healthy self-concepts and modulate aggression. Other groups that deserve further study, as possible problems in object constancy, are certain school phobias and the masochistic stance of some anorexia nervosa patients.

The topic of disorders of object constancy warrants much more extensive consideration. For instance, Akhtar's clinical cases on optimal distance in Chapter 2 raise several interesting questions regarding the similarity and dissimilarity between the disorders of optimal distance and the disorders of object constancy. Are problems in optimal distance more closely related to separation issues and problems in object constancy to individuation issues? Are disorders of object constancy more characteristic of early trauma than conflicts?

When we consider the conflict aspect of Dr. Frank's patient, the centrality of her characterological structure becomes increasingly evident. These traits appear organized around her depressive-masochistic personality (Kernberg 1988).[2] From this vantage point and with the help of the ample clinical material presented by Dr. Frank, we should be able to examine aspects of her masochism from the framework of separation–individuation. Prior to that, however, I would like to raise some questions about Dr. Frank's reconstruction of his case and, as a brief digression, explore his interest in reconstruction.

EARLY TRAUMA AND ITS RECONSTRUCTION

Dr. Frank appears to have separated his patient's problems into early (psychic trauma) and later (conflict) ones and formulated two reconstructions. One reconstruction appears organized around the rapprochement subphase of separation–individuation and contains the loosely organized pre-oedipal material. The other appears organized around oedipal material. It is the blending of the two that gives Dr. Frank's case its unique overtones. I was particularly interested in Dr. Frank's use of reconstruction and his tendency to closely interrelate it to the

---

2. Many analysts (e.g., Asch 1988, Kernberg, 1988) comment on the similarity of the dynamics between depression and masochism.

curative process, the topic of his paper for the International Congress on Psychic Change (Frank 1991). One has the sense that along with Valenstein (1980) and Loewald (1957), Dr. Frank finds it important to "experience" the analytic process along with his patients, providing a level of mutual reliving which he describes in terms of being a biographer for the patient. Being a biographer is an interesting metaphor, since it adds a connotation of objectivity to the close mutual working of the analyst with his patient. Dr. Frank (1991) comments that the analyst takes the "integration provided by the comprehensive reconstruction" (p. 25) and uses the experience as an organizing frame of reference to rewrite the patient's "personal myth" (Kris 1956b). In so doing, he not only brings it in line with reality but also provides explanations for the original distortions. Dr. Frank (1991) emphasizes that a reconstruction should provide such a fuller explanation of psychopathology and not merely fill in the gaps caused by repression. Too often in our technique, interpretations serve to provide the stimulus to recover memories but do not offer the integrative network possible with reconstruction.

This resurgence of interest in reconstruction as a major curative instrument was attributed by Valenstein (1980) to the "widening scope of psychoanalysis and the deepening interest in preverbal development" (p. 434). The interest in reconstruction began to wane when Freud launched metapsychology as a science. With the subsequently increased interest in metapsychology and its emphasis on scientific reductionism, reconstruction with its speculative nature and lack of scientific objectivity fell into dispute (Greenacre 1981, p. 31). The metapsychological bent of the theory led to the opinion that fantasy and not trauma was the etiological agent in neurosis. Trauma was relegated to a secondary role, that is, as a stimulus for fantasy. The recently revived interest in reconstruction has restimulated our interest in trauma as well.

With these considerations in mind, we are in a position to consider the structural defects that Dr. Frank labeled "incapacities" in his patient. Dr. Frank's reconstructions, as is typical of most reconstructions in adult analysis, begin with the latter part of the second year of life of his patient. It is at this crossroad, roughly coinciding with the rapprochement subphase, that the trauma from even earlier stages of development are consolidated. At this time, the preverbal forms of expression (e.g., gesturing, primitive affects, and somatization) and the partially internalized objects are amalgamated with early verbal productions. It is from the vast reservoir of the "unrememberable and unforgettable" (Frank 1969) that these productions are drawn. Their consolidation is made possible by the increasing ascension of the integrative function of the ego over its defensive function (Loewald 1951). One of the results of this activity is that the child discovers that he can create his "own reality" (Lester 1983, Rubinfine 1961). Not surprisingly, "personal myths" (Kris 1956b) frequently have their beginning at this stage.

In reviewing the early infantile material and the second year of life of Dr. Frank's patient, three general areas of trauma should be kept in mind:

1. The most frequently encountered trauma in the reconstructed cases of adult analysis is the strain trauma (Kris 1956), that is, longstanding frustrations that are the result of accumulative trauma as opposed to a singular acute incident or the shock trauma.
2. Sandler's (1987) concept of screen trauma seems applicable when considering the patient's use of the domestic couple in her "personal myth" as a screen function to cover the first year of life. Screen traumas often have a defensive function, particularly when the function involves a "shifting of guilt" for forbidden sexual or aggressive impulses (Sandler 1962).
3. Hoffer's (1952) concept of silent trauma appears to hold particular importance in understanding the patient's aversion to the couch and the transient loss of reality

without visual contact with the analyst. Such occurrences are "more characteristic for the undifferentiated state of the id–ego relationship than later stages of ego development." [p. 38]

Early developmental failures, that is, less than optimal passage through the symbiotic phase of development, can have far-reaching implications for subsequent development of body image and for the establishment of self-boundaries. Weil (1985) described the symptom formations that can occur in the future as a result of a less than optimal symbiotic phase. These include attachment to pain, the masochistic character, a propensity toward negative therapeutic reaction, a basic depressive response, and generalized anhedonia. Her concept of the "basic core" (Weil 1970) is also relevant here. It is at the height of the symbiotic phase that the basic core becomes discernible, but it is in the rapprochement subphase that later psychopathology is superimposed and intertwined with the basic core. In brief, a "preponderance of the aggressive drive components, enhanced by a high potential or by early distress caused by a failure in the symbiotic phase, may lead to early deviational base with which neurotic development may amalgamate at later stages of development" (Weil 1985, p. 343).

MASOCHISM AND UNRESOLVED SEPARATION-INDIVIDUATION

One is also impressed by the narcissistic and masochistic qualities of the patient's struggle to control the analyst and the analysis. This struggle gives the material an unmistakable flavor of the rapprochement crisis. These characterological conflicts may best be viewed clinically as dealing with depression and masochism. Kernberg (1988) described the depressive masochistic personality organization as the most common "higher-order" neurotic character organization among the masochistic group. As might be anticipated, the patient's conflicts are laid out and understood most clearly in the transference. Here, her overdependency on support, love, and acceptance from others (especially the analyst), her problems with a severe superego, and her difficulties with aggression are most evident. Many of these traits are common to moral masochism. In particular, we can now regard the boundaries of masochism as involving normal and pathological narcissism. It is therefore not surprising that some of the patient's more pathological problems betrayed the need both to control and to cling. In regard to the drives, her use of sexuality as a defense against her self-destructive impulses was especially evident in the termination phase. That is, aggression was recruited into the service of her eroticism. Gratification was obtained from the sense that she was being improperly treated, causing her to deal with the analyst as if she were morally superior to him. Her enactments within the analysis were not to obtain libidinal gratification but to confirm that such gratification was not available.

Kernberg discussed the pre-oedipal determinants in masochism but placed the dynamics around the oedipal conflict. Cooper (1988), writing on masochism, did not ascribe to the centrality of the Oedipus, although he acknowledged that pre-oedipal issues are reworked through the Oedipus. For Cooper, masochistic defenses ubiquitously arise in the pre-oedipal narcissistic development. He argued strongly for the concept of a single character type—the "narcissistic-masochistic character"—rather than two separate entities.

From the vantage point of separation–individuation theory, masochism has its beginnings within the basic core and with a less than optimal passage through the symbiotic phase. The pleasure in unpleasure exists as an inborn tendency, which makes it easy and inevitable for its development and which occurs at the earliest stages of object differentiation (Bergler 1949). Hoffer (1952) noted the intense oral-sadistic pressure infants struggle against and stressed the importance of pain in regulating the infants' responses to this pressure. The preponderance of aggressive drive becomes pivotal in the mounting aberrant and deviant behavior that encompasses future masochistic traits. Finally, this pleasure in unpleasure becomes consolidated in "the disappointing realization of the helplessness during the rapprochement subphase of separation–individuation" (Cooper 1988, p. 122). Herman (1976) succinctly captured the role of unresolved separation–individuation in masochism when he conceptualized masochism as the failure of successfully separating with a reactive repetition of separation trauma.

The extent and depth of Dr. Frank's patient's self-destructive acting out can be seen in the termination material and in her control of termination. The patient's tears at the time of termination can be seen as a reliving of a preverbal experience. However, her tears may represent not only aspects of the mourning process but also her inconsolability, an expression itself of her profound self-destructiveness. That is, the irreconcilable conflicts within the transference may have become too destructive for the patient to deal with further, precipitating her need to move toward termination. Reenactment in this preverbal experience could then be seen as the realization that she had no capacity to comfort herself and her imperative need to induce a caretaker (the analyst) to effectively comfort her had failed. A sad but still prevailing attitude of control was her only resolution. It permitted her to deny gratification and remove the analyst from her mind. (Her resolution of the termination phase appears similar to one of my patients who deals with her children's summer departure to camp by removing all pictures, clothing, and so on, and placing them in a locked room. As long as there are no reminders of the children, she deals well with their departure.)

ARCHAIC TRANSFERENCES

The structural defect expressed in the inability of the patient to use the couch permits us to consider some archaic transferences.

When considering the transference and countertransference reaction in Dr. Frank's case, I was reminded of certain remarks of Greenson (1988) and Glover (1965). Greenson (1981, p. 209) stated that with some patients, he began the analysis as a "symbiotic self-object," then moved to become a "transitional object" as the analysis progressed, and at termination became a "real person." Glover (1965) coined the term "floating transferences" to describe those transference reactions that show a quality of "transitional phenomena" with fluid shifts in self--other and inside-outside boundaries. Floating transferences permit more scattering and a rapid deployment of themes while avoiding the "focused" quality seen in more classical transferences. Such transferences are often associated with altered states of consciousness with psychoticlike experiences and with hypnagogic episodes akin to the *pavor nocturnus* syndrome of young children. They are also characterized by an intensity of feelings seen in narcissistic borderline pathology. Dr. Frank describes both of these reactions (rapidity of themes and intensity of affects) as characteristic of his patient.

The capacity of patients to react in a transferential way to an analyst's office and to their analysis rather than to the analyst is commented on by Greenson (1981). Transference reactions to inanimate objects are considered by him to be movement in the area of the transitional object. The couch, its coverings, or something else in the immediate area is frequently treated as a transitional object. The neurotic patient, in contrast, has no difficulty seeing these objects as illusory. The objects may be alternately loved and hated, but they endure and survive. With increasing compromise of reality, transitional objects take on a "delusional" quality of reality that is terrifying (Rosenfeld 1952, Searles 1960). Such experiences lead to disintegration rather than the serving of the integrative function typical of the "neurotic" transitional phenomena.

The clinical material supports Dr. Frank's contentions that the analytic work appeared to take place in the re-created aura of the rapprochement subphase. He cites material that parallels

Galenson and Roiphe's (1980) observational work in the preoedipal boy's passage through the rapprochement subphase. The patient's turning away from the unavailable mother toward the father established strong identification patterns with the father during the separation–individuation process (see the concept of role responsiveness in Sandler 1978). These early patterns were instrumental in shaping the oedipal configuration along more "masculine" lines. One could speculate that the patient experienced an earlier than anticipated discovery of the anatomical sexual differences with early castration anxiety and penis envy (Mahler 1975, p. 192). Such proclivities are heightened in development by the intensity of toilet training and the birth of siblings. These two events coincided in this patient's life. The early positive identification of the child with the father and the dread of the engulfing mother are carried into the Oedipus complex. Even though we are accustomed to regarding castration anxiety as paternal, there is ample evidence throughout the analytic literature to support an earlier, basic component of castration anxiety, namely, "the dread of the vulva" (engulfment), which exists independent of the "dread of the father's penis" (Loewald 1951, pp. 13–15).

There are other aspects of the patient's analysis that give the clinical material the stamp of the rapprochement subphase. Her continuing struggle for control in the analysis is reminiscent of the child in rapprochement crisis. Her struggle to keep from surrendering her libidinal, dependent, needy self to the analyst was characterized by gleeful victory over the analysis. Her use of negativism to defeat the analyst became essential for maintaining her self-esteem. For the patient, gratification was achieved by masochistic pleasure in the ability to control her impulses and others. The sexualization of her hostile, aggressive drives represented an important destructive component to her analysis. Recently, we have tended to "desexualize" our concepts of masochism. The defensive use of sexualization is used masochistically in managing separation, loss, helplessness, and destruction. We also have a tendency to avoid emphasizing the self-destructive quality in masochism in our attempts to separate masochism from the perversions. Masochistic symptoms are less flamboyant than the perversions and more "silently" destructive; by not taking adequate notice of this, we join the masochistic patients in their destructiveness.

CONCLUDING REMARKS

Using Dr. Frank's case, I have considered the contribution of separation–individuation to the masochistic process. We might now consider how pain, that is, pleasure in unpleasure, the core of masochism, influences the separation–individuation process. Cooper (1988), for example, considers pain as a necessary and unavoidable concomitant of separation–individuation. When separation and loss are experienced in the normal separation–individuation process, there is a turning to the outside world that is always perceived as a narcissistic injury. To the degree that pain encountered in separation and loss furthers self-definition, it becomes a dominant force in individuation and autonomy. One might even say that it is through the act of mastery of such pain (i.e., its self-regulation and self-induction) that the satisfaction in having achieved autonomy and endured it is obtained (Cooper 1988).

There are at least two mechanisms whereby pain becomes a critical factor in the separation–individuation process. Kestenberg (1971) believed that each phase of development requires a reformulation of self and object representation that includes shifts in the optimal distance between them. This maintains the integrity and continuity of self–object relations in the separation–individuation process despite the loss. It also regulates the degree of pain and autonomy tolerated. This is accomplished by replacing the former symbiotic bonds with lesser symbiotic bonds or with "bridges" such as body products (the intermediate object), with external possessions [Winnicott's (1953) transitional objects], and/or with people (accessory objects). A second method involves the secondary autonomy of the ego and the "change of function" (Hartmann 1958, p. 25) mechanism, that is, literally turning an evil into a virtue over the course of human development. As Loewald (1960) explained:

> Separation from a love object while in one sense something to be overcome and undone through internalization is, insofar as it means individuation and emancipation, a positive achievement brought about by the relinquishment and internalization of the love object. The change of function taking place here is that a means of defense against the pain and anxiety of separation and loss becomes a goal in itself. [p. 264]

We need only to expand the concept of the loss of a love object to include the lost, abandoned ego ideals that we also must separate from and mourn to combine narcissism with masochism. The pain and anxiety of these separations lead us to conclude that individuation is perhaps never achieved without pain. From the side of the drives, the normal response to pain is aggression directed at the cause of pain. From the side of the ego, however, pain can elicit many responses. One of them, which requires a working through similar to the mourning process, is the achievement of individuation. The story of Dr. Frank's patient is a story of both pain and achievement.

REFERENCES

Asch, S. (1988). The analytic concepts of masochism: a reevaluation. In *Masochism: Current Psychoanalytic Perspectives,* ed. R. Glick and D. Meyers, pp. 93–115. Hillsdale, NJ: The Analytic Press.

Bergler, E. (1949). *The Basic Neurosis, Oral Regression and Psychic Masochism.* New York: Grune & Stratton.

Bouvet, M. (1958). Technical variation and the concept of distance. *International Journal of Psycho-Analysis* 39:211–221.

Cooper, A. (1988). The narcissistic-masochistic character. In *Masochism: Current Psychoanalytic Perspectives*, ed. R. Glick and D. Meyers, pp. 119-137. Hillsdale, NJ: The Analytic Press.
Frank, H. (1969). The unrememberable and the unforgettable: passive primal repression. *Psychoanalytic Study of the Child* 24:48-77. New York: International Universities Press.
——— (1991). Psychic change and the analyst as biographer: transference and reconstruction. *International Journal of Psycho-Analysis* 72:22-26.
Freud, S. (1912). Recommendations to physicians practising psycho-analysis. *Standard Edition* 12:109-120.
Galenson, E., and Roiphe, H. (1980). The preoedipal development of the boy. *Journal of the American Psychoanalytic Association* 28:805-828.
Glover, E. (1965). *The Technique of Psychoanalysis*. New York: International Universities Press.
Greenacre, P. (1981). Reconstruction: its nature and therapeutic value. *Journal of the American Psychoanalytic Association* 29:27-46.
Greenson, R. (1981). On transitional objects and transference. In *Between Reality and Fantasy, Winnicott's Concept of Transitional Objects and Phenomena*, ed. S. Grolnick and L. Barkin, pp. 203-209. Northvale, NJ: Jason Aronson, Inc.
Hartmann, H. (1958). *Ego Psychology and the Problem of Adaptation*. New York: International Universities Press.
Herman, J. (1976). Clinging, going in search. *Psychoanalytic Quarterly* 44:5-36.
Hoffer, W. (1952). The mutual influence in the development of ego and the id: earliest stages. *Psychoanalytic Study of the Child* 7:31-41. New York: International Universities Press.
Kernberg, O. (1988). Clinical dimensions of masochism. In *Masochism: Current Psychoanalytic Perspectives*, ed. R. Glick and D. Meyers, pp. 61-79. Hillsdale, NJ: The Analytic Press.
Kestenberg, J. S. (1971). From organ-object imagery to self and object representations. In *Separation-Individuation: Essays in Honor of Margaret S. Mahler*, ed. J. McDevitt and C. Settlage, pp. 75-99. New York: International Universities Press.
Kramer, S. (1980). Residues of self-object and split-self dichotomies in adolescence. In *Rapprochement: The Critical Subphase of Separation-Individuation*, ed. R. Lax, S. Bach, and A. Burland, pp. 417-438. New York: Jason Aronson.
Kris, E. (1956a). The recovery of childhood memories in psychoanalysis. *Psychoanalytic Study of the Child* 11:54-88. New York: International Universities Press.
——— (1956b). The personal myth. *Journal of the American Psychoanalytic Association* 4:653-681.
Lester, S. (1983). Separation and cognition. *Journal of the American Psychoanalytic Association* 31:127-155.
Loewald, H. (1951). Ego and reality. In *Papers on Psychoanalysis*, pp. 3-20. New Haven: Yale University Press, 1980.
——— (1957). On the therapeutic action of psychoanalysis. In *Papers on Psychoanalysis*, pp. 222-256. New Haven, CT: Yale University Press, 1980.

—— (1960). Internalization: separation, mourning and the superego. In *Papers on Psychoanalysis*, pp. 257–276. New Haven, CT: Yale University Press, 1980.

Mahler, M. S. (1975). On the current status of the infantile neurosis. In *The Selected Papers of Margaret S. Mahler*, vol. 2, pp. 188–193. New York: Jason Aronson, 1982.

—— (1977). Developmental aspects in the assessment of narcissistic and so-called borderline personalities. In *The Selected Papers of Margaret S. Mahler*, vol. 2, pp. 195–209. New York: Jason Aronson, 1982.

Roazen, P. (1975). *Freud and His Followers.* New York: Alfred A. Knopf.

Rosenfeld, H. A. (1952). Transference phenomena and transference analysis in an acute catatonic schizophrenia patient. In *Psychotic States: A Psychoanalytic Approach*, pp. 104–116. New York: International Universities Press, 1965.

Rubinfine, D. (1961). Perception, reality testing and symbolism. *Psychoanalytic Study of the Child* 16:73–89. New York: International Universities Press.

Sandler, J. (1962). Hampstead index as an instrument of psychoanalytic research. *International Journal of Psycho-Analysis* 43:287–291.

—— (1987). *From Safety to Superego: Selected Papers of Joseph Sandler.* New York: Guilford Press.

Sandler, J., and Sandler, A. M. (1978). On the development of object relationships and affects. *International Journal of Psycho-Analysis* 59:285–296.

Searles, H. (1960). *The Non-Human Environment on Normal Development and in Schizophrenia.* New York: International Universities Press.

Valenstein, A. (1980). Preoedipal reconstructions in psychoanalysis. *International Journal of Psycho-Analysis* 70:433–442.

Weil, A. (1970). The basic core. *Psychoanalytic Study of the Child* 25:422–460. New York: International Universities Press.

—— (1985). Thoughts on early pathology. *Journal of the American Psychoanalytic Association* 33:335–352.

Winnicott, D. (1953). Transitional object and transitional phenomena: a case study of the first not-me possessions. In *Collected Papers: Through Pediatrics to Psychoanalysis*, pp. 229–242. London: Tavistock, 1958.

6

NONVERBAL BEHAVIORS IN THE ANALYTIC SITUATION: THE SEARCH FOR MEANING IN NONVERBAL CUES

James T. McLaughlin, M.D.

He that has eyes to see and ears to hear may convince himself that no mortal can keep a secret. If his lips are silent, he chatters with his fingertips; betrayal oozes out of him at every pore. (Freud 1905)

ELOQUENT HANDS

Mr. E. enters my office in his usual fashion, as he has done four times a week since he began to lie on my couch two years ago. A slim, somber man, tight and constrained in body and manner, he strides past me without comment, quickly wiping his nose and mouth with the back of his right hand as he passes me. While his eyes never meet mine, I can see from their oblique set in my direction that he keeps me in his peripheral vision as long as he can. I have had many thoughts about his behavior, each time he has passed. When I saw it for the very first time it made me think of the eyes-right-pass-in-review parades I sweated through in my army days, and his a rather strange salute.

Mr. E. stretches out on the couch in a relaxed fashion, hands laced behind his head, right leg bent and resting on his left leg. He immediately begins telling me about his many successful enterprises, soon gesticulating vigorously in the air with his right hand. His speech is declamatory and at times loud; his voice conveys intensities that I hear as pleasure and pride mixed with some anxiety and pleading. The contrast between off- and on-couch behaviors is striking, even though I have seen it played out like this for the last three months.

There are other contrasts, equally striking, when I think back to his first year on the couch. Then Mr. E. lay stretched out motionlessly, legs side by side, hands clasped tightly on his upper abdomen. His voice was small, and often I had to strain to hear his brief phrases, remarkable in their cautious generalities, constant revisions, and disclaimers. His most frequent expressions were "but, I don't know" as a coda to his own commentary, and "it could be" as a response to mine. My initial appraisal of him was that he was a bright, even intellectually gifted, man, inhibited in assertiveness and lacking in self-esteem, held back in his full unfolding by obsessional defenses against strong affectivity.

Back then, Mr. E. lay very still on the couch. His main motor activity, one that went on almost incessantly from the first couch hour, was his hand play. I cannot recall another patient whose constantly touching hands held so rich a repertory of hand-to-hand combat, play, and lovemaking. His fingertips and nails were tattered survivors of years of picking and tearing that went on in bursts, in a manner I presumed to be a habitual cuticle picking and nibbling habit. At lesser intensity, his fingers scratched, squeezed, tapped, and banged on each other, or, at times, gently smoothed and massaged themselves or those of the other hand. His thumbs had their own place in the action, tapping on or twirling around each other, concealed in the curled fingers of own or opposite hand, and often the target of attack or caress from the other hand.

While we worked together in the first year or so, in an analytic mode wherein I maintained a rather quiet style, I had ample opportunity to observe these hand behaviors as they played out in the context of the verbal component of our dialogue. Mr. E. was one of those patients whom I attempted to track with a style of observing and note taking that I have described elsewhere (McLaughlin 1987). Its essence lay in my trying, with process notes and scrawled gestural notations, to capture in near simultaneity the words and actions of my patient.

The stimulus for this attempt came from experiences that I kept having while watching, largely with left peripheral vision, the kinesic behaviors of my patients as they lay diagonally to my left. What kept happening, without my consciously intending, was that often, as I looked and listened, I experienced a dawning sense of pattern or context relating to the verbal, actional, and affective components of the patient's communication. I did not know what it was that I had registered; but, repeated variously over analytic time, the patterns had become recognizable, even though not yet identifiable. Hence the search for learning what I could about these simultaneities.

Those of you who know this story will remember that the sheer burden it placed on my efforts to analyze forced me to put the project aside except for spot sampling and following change over time. I did find that it was descriptively possible, and clinically useful, to distinguish between behaviors that were occasional, conspicuous, and idiosyncratic and those gestural patterns that were repetitious, unobtrusive, and likely to go unnoticed until repeated over time in synchrony with verbalized content (McLaughlin 1987, pp. 573–577).

In Mr. E.'s case I had no chance to be rigorous, for the rapidity of his hand activities was beyond my capacities to record but a fraction. Yet I did register much, in the multilevel ways of seeing and hearing that we all habitually use, often without our conscious knowing. It is from the sum of what I came to know in this manner about this patient, how he behaved as he spoke of himself and those around him, that I draw in scanning Mr. E.'s behaviors and analytic progress in his first year of analytic work.

I learned that Mr. E. had grown up as the middle child of three, with a sister three years older and a brother who came along just two years later. Both parents struggled to survive in separate professional careers that took them early and often away from the home, once the youngest child was born. My patient carried a blur of memories from his early years of cleaning women and sitters looking in on him and the other two. He had sharper recall in his memories, some of these his earliest, of his turning, as did his brother, to his sister for attention.

He still felt grateful to his sister for what she provided, although it came in ways imitative of his mother's unreliable bursts of caring. In our work he tended to merge mother and sister in his sortings of his past. He described both as being at times solicitous and doing for him, in ways that could be comforting, yet more often taking him over and doing *to* him while demanding his grateful compliance. Both were capricious and totally unpredictable in responding or ignoring; either could turn on him with fury, slaps, and stomping off, if what he did offended her. He remembered being bewildered and upset, lost and helpless, growing quiet and cautious.

A parallel but very different confluence showed in his perceptions of brother and father. Mr. E. lumped them together with tolerant dismissal. Brother was more bother than he was worth, someone to team up with in warding off, baiting, or competing with big sister; an uncertain ally in a show of strength in standing up to mother's absolute power, and another loser in their conviction that mother vastly preferred their sister. Mr. E. had vague guilt over having distanced himself early from his brother's littleness and haplessness, and watching with disdain his brother's floundering even in adulthood. Father was portrayed from a position of distance and uncertainty. Mr. E. was his most indecisive and noncommittal in letting me know about his father, who came across as someone absorbed in his own struggles to cope with life in general, his wife in particular, as a nonpresence in relation to any of his children. When the father did get involved with the two boys, he did so through perfunctory disciplining demanded by the mother. The two boys shared the conviction that the father, too, preferred their self-assured and colorful sister.

I will sample in summary fashion some of the rich concurrence that I often saw, and occasionally recorded, between Mr. E.'s hand/finger play and his verbal/affective associations around these central figures of his primary family. Much of this kinesic patterning became active when he was caught up in thinking about his wife and others of importance to his current life and, in time, about me. I shall refer to these collateral happenings mainly to instance their transference implications. I could see no indication that any of these small behaviors were in the patient's awareness.

Soon into the analysis Mr. E. altered his basic clasped-hands position in different ways and in different contexts. When he spoke of needing comforting or reassurance from his wife, then associatively his sister, the fingers of his left hand might free themselves to cover, and gently rub, the back of his right hand. Then his thumb, usually the right, could slowly be enfolded in the clasp of the other hand. He did not make this kinesic linkage when speaking of his mother. Toward her he described more his wariness of never knowing whether she would remain calm or overwhelm him in unprovoked verbal and physical assault. Here one thumb would rapidly disappear into the clasp of the other hand or of its fellow fingers; in a frequent variant, both thumbs could tuck out of sight beneath the still-interlocked fingers. From his words I began to hear a richer context for his troubles with the mother as these small rituals played on. His mother had pressed him to be a big boy in complying quickly with her rules about obedience, sphincter control, and eating what was put before him. At the same time, she could not tolerate his efforts to do things his way and became angry, often physically punitive, at his willfulness, his straying away, and his curiosity about her body and that of the woman caretakers who came and went. He had been provocative briefly but had crumpled into overt submission out of fear of banishment. As he grew, he became stubborn and subversive, never capitulating completely.

As he slowly became freer to reveal himself to me, in what I sensed to be a form of idealizing transference, he drummed on the back of one hand with the stiffened fingers of the other, back and forth, with great vigor and audible force. Mainly he spoke at such times of his controlled anger at his mother for the constraints she had placed upon him, his rage toward her that he felt helpless to express lest she retaliate tenfold. His heightened body tension amplified the anxiety engendered in him as he spoke of how it was to this day when in any way he was stirred to anger by anyone important to him. The finger drumming also began to occur during silences between us. We could explore these silences gradually, and he could acknowledge that he perceived my silences as failing to meet his silent needing that I help him to deal better with his emerging rage toward his mother.

It was around this time, toward the end of his first year in analysis, that his thumb picking stepped up in tempo and prominence. Able to speak more fully of his needs and frustrations felt in relation to both parents, and now toward me, he began openly to pick at the skin of both thumbs with thumb and index finger of the other hand. These attacks were at times literally bloody. This prompted me, for the first time, to call direct attention to these kinesics, partly out of mild concern for this self-mutilating, partly because I knew from my analytic explorations of my own adolescent cuticle picking what rich dynamics of pent-up anger and sexual conflict could lie in this behavior. Finally, I assumed that the pain he was experiencing must surely be in his awareness.

I was wrong in my assumption. Mr. E. showed shock, anxiety, and speechlessness. Later he described his silence as first a fear of saying anything at all, then a state of confusion and fear.

At that moment of his confusion I intervened actively to reflect upon his apparent state and how what I had done had upset him so. Gradually he regrouped and spoke of being entirely unaware of his skin picking; he felt caught and about to be given a beating, or told he was unanalyzable and we were through. He acknowledged that his cuticle picking was a habit from his early school years, but he had nothing more to say at that point. Following our enactment, this kinesic pattern left the analytic scene for several months, although his thumbs, and fingers as well, bore mute witness to ongoing combat elsewhere. Only some months later, as he worked over his experiencing me as having let him down, turned on him, and changed inexplicably from the comforting helper that he thought he had, did more history about these kinesics emerge. Notably, his usual disclaimers and qualifiers had dropped in frequency as this piece of work was accomplished, and he was more forthright in his speaking. He could not remember when his nail biting and picking had begun. It had driven his mother to enraged screaming and face slapping in her helplessness that she could not break him of the habit. He could recall gloves tied on his hands, foul-tasting stuff smeared on his fingers, and beatings given him by both parents. These memories were entangled in other recallings of even earlier battles and chemical warfare around thumb sucking, which struggles his mother apparently had won. This later battle she could not win.

I reflected to him, and he acknowledged, his pride in his nearly lifelong angry, stubborn holding on to what he could that was his own, often at the cost of mutuality and intimacy. Having this struggle played out between us opened the way for us to work on what we both had come to see: the battle scars from both campaigns that left him wary of his wife's often generous giving and my efforts to reach him, his striving to control his temper and his need to overeat, and his guilt over whether he really loved anyone. Then we could address, in conflict terms, the enduring pain of his unmet hopes for steady caring and the anxious fury over the uncertainties of care given or denied.

This samples the manner of our working, up to the state and place where I introduced Mr. E. to the reader. By that time he had shown considerable loosening of his behavioral constriction on the analytic couch, as well as gaining of a broader range of affective freedom and access to aspects of his troubled past that he had repressed earlier or had disavowed. His limited behavioral display had given way gradually to freer kinesics that I inferred, and he corroborated, to be a reflection of his greater comfort and collaborative involvement in the analytic search.

At no time, except for the confrontation I made about the bloody skin tearing, was it necessary to address the hand kinesics directly. The nonverbal components served mainly as guide and affirmation for my enhanced understanding of Mr. E.'s dynamics. These cues often alerted me to his underlying affective states and conflicts at a time when he could not, and would not, put words to them. The metaphor they provided helped me find good words.

He and I had later to do considerable work on castration-level conflicts centered on his avoidance of intellectual aspiration and professional achievement, considered by the patient to be destructively competitive toward both parents and me. Fresh reflection of what turned out to be castration anxiety over exhibiting emerged in a new mannerism of clutching his necktie as he spoke of his desires to excel as an intellect. This conspicuous behavior was one that I could more freely address, in contrast to the quieter background kinesics. After some time I asked him to notice his tight grasping, as something to explore. We learned first that there was an ongoing battle between Mr. E. and his wife about who was to select the ties that he wore. When he wore those that he had chosen, he felt conspicuous and vulnerable to criticism. And well he might, for his were wildly polychrome, hers subdued and sincere. This led him to his choice of a spouse: he had defended against his richly incestuous desires by his lesser marital choice of a sister figure. With her he could gain the comfort of a subtle devaluation of both wife and himself that sidestepped the tensions of his reaching for full revenge and fulfillment. As these old dynamic issues became revived in the analytic work, Mr. E.'s grabbing of his flamboyant ties, at the height of uncertainty over the outcome of his dilemma over wish and fear of accomplishment, made these tensions manifest. Here was something simultaneously real and symbolic that we both could see, grasp, and soon chuckle about, an insight gained between us with a graphic power that words alone could never reach.

At this point we must remain uncertain as to whether these clinical data have demonstrated their relevance for the issues of separation, individuation, and rapprochement that Margaret Mahler and colleagues (1975) helped us see through their infant research. I think that the circumstantial evidence is rather compelling, given its fairly clear linkage to very early dynamic concerns. I shall return to this challenge later.

Meanwhile, I want to stress that a particular reason for providing this overview has been to describe the changes that can be discerned in the background kinesics of a not-extraordinary analytic patient as the work progressed. These changes that patients generally experience as they improve over analytic time are much like those described for Mr. E.: the gradual relinquishment of initial constraint and prevailing immobility, and the achievement of evident relaxation and more freely displayed expressive motility. The initial background kinesics tend to drop away in frequency as the accompanying dynamic concerns are reduced through the analytic work, resurfacing occasionally as these concerns return for further working through. I have found these changes particularly in those patients with a preponderance of inhibitory neurotic symptoms and obsessional character disposition.

RESTLESS FEET

My second vignette is more immediate in its clinical detail and more graphic in its depiction of uncertain object constancy. It may be more compelling in its portrayal of linkage between verified experiences of specific traumata occurring in the first two years of life and separation–individuation dynamics played out in the patient's behaviors as an adult.

Mrs. T. presents a quite different picture and clinical challenge than Mr. E., at a time when she is well into the third year of an increasingly turbulent analysis.[1] Thanks to repeated small enactments of our shared shaping, we are having growing difficulty in working without encountering another troublesome break in our communication.

Mrs. T. enters grim-faced and flashes a brief blank stare in passing. The following dialogue illustrates our interaction at the time:

> *Mrs. T.* I thought what you had to say on Friday was crap, way off target; left me nowhere all weekend. Made me think of other stuff like it you've said that was just as off the wall. Can't remember what it was. (Right hand clutches strands of gold necklace on upper chest.) Can you?
>
> *A.* Maybe you can get to it. We can see—
>
> *Mrs. T.* Not much help, as usual—something about how I don't pay attention to what you say, can't let you help me. Which is a crock. I ask your help and you don't even *hear*. And that stuff last week about how my mother conned me into dumping my bottle in the trash can, said be a big girl; and I wasn't ready to give her *it,* I mean, up. You acting like that meant something, and I don't think it meant much! (Right hand flings chain with motion that bounces necklace off her nose and lips as she gesticulates to right, toward me. Pause. Near crying.) Why don't you help me!

---

1. She, like Mr. E., was one of those patients with whom I attempted to capture the simultaneity of verbal and kinesic content. These clinical data were presented on October 5, 1982, as part of a panel presentation of the Workshop Series of the American Psychoanalytic Association entitled "The Relevance of Infant Observational Research for Clinical Work with Adults." Reference to Mrs. T. also in McLaughlin (1987).

(Right hand clutching and twisting chain on her throat.) I could choke you!

A. How do you see my helping you?

Mrs. T. See! You don't even know! You're not paying attention. You *should* know, and why should I have to tell you, come to you? Why aren't you *there?* (Hands clutch each other on chest.) It's no use. I'm always on my own, floundering. Trying to learn how to feel good feelings, to relax and feel my sexual feelings; instead, just tighten up, get anxious; then feel nothing but anxiety and anger everywhere. I leave here like this and go out there and get into real trouble, lose my job, my home, my chance to have a baby, have my feelings! *Say* something! (Voice in high-pitched anxious rage; right hand clutches necklace, left fingers to mouth.)

A. Perhaps we can look at your getting afraid here when you try to feel good. Something happens in you that you have to stop the good feelings, become empty and frustrated.

Mrs. E. (After long silence, then in cold contempt and fury, hands pounding the couch.) *That* does it! That ruins *this* hour! I ask your help in letting me feel good, relaxed, and right, and you tell me to go be afraid of you, tighten up; rub my nose in it and there's nothing there! I could claw you, rip off your genitals, break up this room! (Sits up to glare at me and kicks at the coffee table. Long, silent glaring.)

A. Are you thinking of something?

Mrs. T. (Still furious.) I am but I won't! Talking about what you want talked about will just push me down deeper into the muck. I could just walk out of here and never come back—or come back with my gun!

A. You see me as making you do what I want, go look in the garbage can for what isn't there?

(Pause)

Mrs. T. You bastard; you're doing just what you were doing on Friday, rubbing my nose in how much I need you and can't do without you or *with* you. (Quieting a bit, still glaring, right hand clutching necklace almost to breaking point.) You keep *doing* this to me; just when I'm going to risk letting you see me being me, you're off somewhere or telling me I ought to be looking at something else, or go lie on the couch all by myself! (Silence of several minutes of near-unblinking staring at me, as I look wide-eyed back, leaning forward in my chair a little. She breaks gaze and swings round so as to be half-sprawled away from me, face muffled in the couch; mumbles inaudibly.)

A. (Leaning forward in chair) I'm sorry. I just can't hear what you're saying; but it sounds like you're crying.

Mrs. T. If I'm crying it's not for *you,* it's for me. I feel lost and stuck, afraid to get up and get out of here, or what to do if I do. But I'm so goddamned attached to you! (Hand again clutching necklace and blouse at throat.) Why don't you *do* something! (Said with less heat.)

A. Maybe you're saying, "Help me help myself, and stop getting in my way?" (Long silence, perhaps four to five minutes, patient sinking back onto the couch in semi-reclining position, right foot on floor, left hand on forehead, right hand holding necklace and bodice in relaxed way.)

Mrs. T. I'm remembering what you said a long time ago. It wasn't the way I thought you said; had to do with me telling you about that time in the department store and I wanted to look around and [my mother] stood there, let me run off and be lost, and they brought me back crying and I wet myself. You said then that I wasn't letting myself feel anything as I was telling you, and I wouldn't. And you said it was important and I didn't think so. You took it away from me; saw more in it than I did. I couldn't work with it anymore, it wasn't *mine.* But there *was* more to it: she told the clerk she had kept an eye on me all the time; that she wanted me to feel what it was like not to heed and run off and get lost. Years later she told me the same thing and I asked her if it was true. She let me do what I was doing by myself and made it hers, made it bad, to teach me a lesson! Well, she taught me, and I'm all fucked up for it! (Jerking and twisting the necklace, grabbing it and throwing it away in rapid alternation.) Just like she talked me into how good it was to throw away my bottle, and I did, and I didn't feel good at all—I felt lost. And I *did* go looking all over for it, in the garbage can the next day, but it was gone, and I felt gone. (Hands down to sides in opened fashion.) I'm still tied to her, and now I'm stuck to you. (Both hands, white knuckled, clasp necklace.) I want to be on top and instead I'm in the pits. (Pause) You're awfully quiet. Are you there? THERE? (Looks back briefly.) Yeah, guess you are. You usually are. Now, what do I do with that! Maybe you *don't* always crowd me, or leave me like I think. But, it's hard to know you're mine or I'm yours, to count on where I can feel you with me okay.

I think this exchange tells much about the dynamic conflicts and their developmental phase origins of this patient, about whom I have told you practically nothing, as well as about my own, often ill-advised, efforts to make contact with her. I have presented this in its stark and painful actuality in order to ask, as well as to challenge, the reader to resonate to the nonverbal pantomime that complements the verbal communication. At this point in the clinical narrative, I would wonder what you feel can legitimately be inferred, from this single interview alone, about separation, individuation, rapprochement, and transitional phenomena.

Meanwhile, here are some salient aspects about Mrs. T.'s background and a sketch of the course of the analysis up to the time of the interview just described.

> Mrs. T. had entered analysis frantic for help with her worried absorption in her job, her near-disabling anxiety over how she was perceived and treated in her work, her frigidity in her marriage, and her pervasive inability to sustain pleasurable feelings connected with idleness, recreation, or sexuality.
>
> An attractive woman in her late twenties, Mrs. T. struggled to maintain her place in a professional field long known to be dominated by men. She held to firm convictions that any revealing of inadequacy on her part to her male associates would lead to her downfall, and she saw being casually friendly or flirtatious as a bow to their chauvinism that left her shamed and guilty. In actuality, she continually encountered what she feared, both with her bosses and her husband. Her accounts of being "put down" by all those in power portrayed her as behaving habitually in a muted, self-depreciative way until goaded to

petulant complaining that provoked further rejection. Her manner of relating to me gradually portrayed this pattern. At the beginning she was eager to please and anxiously bent on avoiding my criticism. I often had to strain to hear her small voice or decipher her quick, slurred words. My asking her to repeat or clarify brought her to flushed confusion and stammering, and she acknowledged that she felt criticized and uptight.

Initially compliant and clinging to my words as gospel, Mrs. T. spun out her story of sturdily trying to ward off disasters that still kept happening. She gradually showed flashes of tense playfulness, at times being provocatively flirtatious. When I kept failing to respond, except to inquire further, she became abashed, ashamed, and angrily withdrawn. She initially rebounded to a stance of insistent independence, saying, "Who needs you, anyhow?" Soon she began to subside into a "help me—I don't know what's wrong; what's happening to me?" mode whose evident suffering I experienced poignantly as a pleading to be rescued. I reflected this to her in an exploring and tentative fashion. It was then that I first heard about a chronic illness, during the patient's second five years, that kept her closely dependent upon her mother, whom Mrs. T. described as being then a hovering and solicitous homemaker until the patient's kindergarten years. At that point mother ceased to be housebound and went off to work as a secretary in an office, where she described herself as forever overworked and underappreciated and more burdened than ever at home, but obviously pleased with her career.

Once, as she dwelt wistfully upon those early years of her mother's caring, I could hear Mrs. T.'s gut rumblings, mostly soft gurglings, as she lay quietly, her hands intertwined on her epigastrium. I was first surprised, and a bit abashed, when I heard *my* gut sounds, piping a kind of counterpoint, or obligato, to hers. Mrs. T. also heard, and she reacted alertly. "Are you making that sound to tease me, like at times the tapes you play in the sun porch seem like you chose them on purpose?" While I was pondering an answer, my gut obligingly rumbled again. This time, Mrs. T. laughed in what seemed to me relief (hers, or mine?) and said: "Well, I guess I finally got a response out of you!" Later, as she reminisced about instances of her mother's solicitude whenever the patient was hurting, and her stomach would speak, she seemed to be listening for me to repeat my contribution to the duet. When on occasion this did happen and I silently resigned, she spoke with pleasure about how this "seemed to bring us close, like we were joined." I may have been acting analytically, but I do know that I felt some anxious press to reclaim the right to speak for myself when I acknowledged that we both seemed to find some special meaning in the images of a caring mother being close to her hurting child.

Shortly afterward Mrs. T. began, for the first time, to cry in my presence, as she related aspects of her early years that cast her mother in a different light than the rosy idealizing of her initial account of her childhood.

Haltingly, Mrs. T. sketched a picture of arriving as the third child of overworked, blue-collar parents absorbed in jobs and home renovations, and eager to speed the maturing of their trio. Only the firstborn, a son, was allowed freedom and the privilege of being with the father in his building projects. The two girls, just eleven months apart, were kept on a short tether and pressed into housekeeping chores that the brother escaped.

Both from her own retrieval of early memories and from family accounts, Mrs. T. had been rushed through weaning from breast and bottle, and toilet trained very early. She had been twinned to her sister by her mother, who dressed and treated them alike for the first six years, pressing both to strict rules of controlled behavior. Her earliest memories were of wrangles with her sister, who would scorn her for her shameful baby weaknesses, then tell on her; of her house-frazzled mother reproving her for bothering everyone with her helpless screaming about unfair treatment.

Mrs. T. had matured early into a good and conscientious little girl who developed in preadolescence a severe religious scrupulosity that caricatured the strict upbringing of home and religious education. In both contexts she was castigated for her sneaky stubbornness and punished for her rare outflares of verbal rebellion; she became guilty and anxious thereafter if she deviated from compliance.

Inwardly chafing over the preferential treatment accorded her brother in furthering his access to sports and education, she experienced rebuff and censure from the parents when she begged for equal opportunity. Instead, she found her own funding for advanced schooling and pushed herself far beyond the levels achieved by parents or siblings. The higher she went, the greater became her anxiety and guilt. She felt estranged and lost in her college years. While in school she quickly entered into marriage to an undemonstrative man, educationally beneath her and given to controlling her with unremitting criticisms and needling of her weaknesses. She was painfully dependent upon his approval, unable to defend herself, and only rarely orgasmic.

To go back again to the beginning of the analysis: Mrs. T. showed from the start an anxious vigilance, gazing intently into my eyes while entering and leaving my office, at times with warm friendliness, at times with baleful glare. On leaving, she invariably said goodbye to me twice, breaking gaze, then quickly looking back to make eye contact again and repeat her farewell. I had a strong sense of being checked upon in her way of being sure that I was still watching. She was visibly uneasy on the couch, finding it hard to lie still, and soon established a behavior of quickly glancing over her right shoulder to make sure I was there. She acknowledged that she needed to check out my facial expressions to see if I were still kindly inclined. She was particularly apt to do so while telling of her sexual and hostile feelings.

Often her anxiety in this regard was such that she would swing suddenly to a sitting posture on the couch, speaking of her need "to feel the floor under my feet." I found that my encouraging her to lie down when she could, for the usual good analytic reasons, evoked only dull submission and affectless rumination, then mute rage and anxiety that we could not work on. Similarly, when I met her sitting gaze with exploring questions and requests for analytic work, her agitation and motility increased. She could not sit but would leap up and rush to the windows at the far end of my office and drum on the panes, or head for the door and stand irresolutely in the doorway, peering intently at my face. If I asked anything of her then or tried to interpret what I thought to be the basis for her turmoil, she was given to quitting the hour entirely. Then later I would hear of more work anxiety, wrangles with husband, hurting her body by stumbling and other kinetic clumsiness, and increased drinking.

Gradually, at these times of her fight or flight, I saw that I did best if I just sat still and returned her gaze with widened eyes and a smiling-inquiring look. Then she would settle down and return to the couch to resume work in her own fashion.

In the context of these anxious activities a most unusual act of postural kinesics came to the fore. While still lying down, Mrs. T. would speak in mounting tension of feeling uptight, helpless, and stuck. Suddenly she would draw her knees upward and flex them so that both feet were flat on the couch. She brought her hands to her shoes, then hooked both forefingers around the heels. As she did this, she spoke anxiously of her fears that she might seduce me, or that I was about to attack her genitals, penetrate her sexually. Then she would be irreparably damaged; mother would discover and banish patient forever from her sight. An alternative outcome, exciting but sure to leave her deserted and guilty, was that I would claim her and force her to sex and elopement. I was struck at such times that Mrs. T. did not seem to own her body or her sexuality; she appeared helplessly ready to allow them to be at the whim of any forceful man.

I watched this combination of kinesics and content for a few months, exploring the latter but not addressing the odd kinesic display. The yield was meager. I called attention to her hold on her heels and asked her what it felt like, or made her think of. She obviously felt caught, released her heels, and brought her legs down to stretch; said she was very uptight. I agreed that I could hear her distress and said I really wasn't expecting any answer unless she found something in it that she would want to work on. This she eventually did, in her way. First, she casually informed me that she had suffered from a chronic urinary tract problem, from age 6 to 14. The details gradually emerged. She had been made to lie still for many urological exams and procedures, often prolonged and painful, on her back and in stirrups. She tried to heed the demands of the male urologists that she be a good girl, to lie still and be quiet. She did her best, with held-in rebellion and fear. As she reworked this recall with tears and muted anger, she retrieved memories of frequent genital stirrings and erotic interest in some of the doctors. She recalled both feeling ashamed and frightened that her excitement might show, as well as defiant protest that it was not her fault the doctors wanted to do these things to her. For some time, working over this stretch of traumatic history allowed her to settle in upon the couch more comfortably.

During this time of relative comfort I watched Mrs. T. bring into play this stirrup posture in synchrony with a very different verbal content. She reached for her heels often when speaking of her conflicted wishes to assert her independence of her mother. She saw mother as binding her by somehow filling Mrs. T. with guilt over any emotional distancing from mother, or being different from mother over the right ways for their relating to each other. She "wanted so much to be my own self, free to fly!" and held her heels. Her pain over differences had spread to include feeling disloyal for any enjoyment of the pleasures of living, including sex, that she felt her mother did not enjoy or endorse. Mrs. T. could allow herself very little sense of her own competence in work or play and constricted her intellectual and professional capacities to the point of jeopardy. She did so out of a conscious conviction that to do otherwise was to inflict crushing shame upon her mother and invite the latter's complete rejection and abandonment. Thinking, during an analytic hour, of such a breach between them could bring Mrs. T. to what seemed like near-fragmentation, clutching her heels and quivering. She had long ago learned to restore herself by getting in telephone contact with her mother, to detail her sufferings of the moment, to emphasize to her mother her own helplessness and need for warm reassurance. She had long noticed, but had only now begun to reflect upon, her mother's reliable interest in and consoling response to expressed suffering, yet her notable turning off when Mrs. T. spoke of achievements, travel plans, or free spending.

By the time of the clinical sampling presented above, Mrs. T. was well into her version of a transference neurosis, playing out many of these mother-centered wishes and fears increasingly in her relationship to me. These she phrased mainly in terms of complaints about not getting the relief from anxiety she demanded that I provide for her. She was by now oscillating between rage and rebellion, then compliant beseeching; between tender and timid little-girl amorous overtures and near-belligerent sexual provocativeness. She spoke of fear of sexual attack and genital mutilation by me as real and imminent, but also as irrational fantasy. She was not in touch with her huge envy and strivings to preempt that were aimed toward me as someone combining the life and death powers over her that she attributed both to her mother and to powerful male figures, exemplified by doctors.

While Mrs. T. was usually able to recover her poise and adult perspective on these in-hour preoccupations, I heard increasing complaint of her falling into anxiety states and depression outside the hours and her resorting to wine in the evenings to soothe herself. It took much focusing upon these episodes to learn that they tended to happen when she left an hour in a state of angry distancing from me over some break of comfortable rapport between us. Then she found herself "feeling alone, adrift, not able to think of anything you had said or done, and no pictures of you or the sound of your voice," unlike her comforting recall of me experienced when we were early in the work.

These breakdowns between us often were triggered by certain behaviors of mine as I tried to meet and understand her quicksilver challenges and pleas for rescue or guidance. If I responded in a fashion that carried even a hint of steering or persuading, Mrs. T. could sit up, or leap from the couch, to confront me in blazing-eyed rage, screaming that I had wiped her out, taken her over, and threatening to kill me with some object snatched from the coffee table. If I remained silent, she persisted in her pleadings, then collapsed in a heap, sobbing inconsolably. I found that I could best restore something between us at such times by facing her fury with as much show of relaxed calm as I could muster and talking through her withdrawn sobbing, using slow, quiet words to acknowledge her misery.

This is how things were at the time of the analytic hour with which I prefaced this vignette. We accomplished a lot up to and beyond that hour, the work extending over many years, but we could not go as far as either of us would have liked. Mrs. T. survived family deaths and disasters in solid fashion. Her affect storms largely left the scene, along with her stirrup ritual, but never entirely. Her sexual inhibitions released, and she went on to have two children whose rearing imposed further burdens and seriously curtailed her professional advancement. These combined constraints eventually forced us to drop back to weekly psychotherapy, within whose limitations further working out of her ambivalent dependency and shaky object constancy became protracted.

DISCUSSION

The place and importance of the nonverbal components of the psychoanalytic dialogue have been variably and uncertainly regarded in mainstream psychoanalysis. Analytic pioneers from the beginning addressed, out of clinical necessity and in their fascination with hysterical symptoms, the complexities of the behavioral dance and somatic music that accompany the poetry of human communication. Some became enthralled with the vast significance they found (Groddeck 1928). Others, like Ferenczi (1919), wrestled with the muscular and gut power of what caught them up, and went off in directions of their own in their struggles to acknowledge the role of the nonverbal aspects of their analytic experience.

But what carried the greater weight of persuasion, from the beginnings of analysis to this day, was Freud's overriding commitment to the saving power of rationality and to the secondary processes that language provided to ensure the dominance of reason in human endeavors. This conviction led him, both in his theoretical and in his clinical pronouncements (Freud 1911, 1912, 1913, 1914), to relegate to infantile beginnings and psychic primitivism such matters as body language and organ music. These were to be regarded as the primary stuff, the basic body-ego (Freud 1923), out of which rational man, now epitomized by the generic analyst and the well-analyzed patient, was to shape and assert his higher reality view.

Many enduring perspectives were reached from this vantage point. We still accept as valid the proposition that adult thinking is blended from three essential ingredients: a sensori-motor-visceral-affective mix that is the infant's earliest mode of responding; his later, or perhaps simultaneous, imaging in all sensory modes; and gradually, as childhood is traversed, a verbal-lexical capability that achieves a relative dominance over human behavior (Horowitz 1978). Much that ego psychology has laid out about the emergence of the sense of self, pari passu with the acquisition of operational competence to survive in the world of one's culture, has built upon this hierarchical sequence over which language is king.

We analysts still ascribe central importance to the spoken word as a prime carrier of our therapeutic endeavors, even though we may no longer agree with the rigors of Eissler's (1953) technical distinctions regarding what is, or what is not, truly psychoanalysis. A major liability, however, in this emphasis upon the primacy of the spoken word has lain in a pervasive tendency among us to look upon the nonverbal components generally as an inferior and lower-order capability, a marker of the infantile and regressed, in keeping with other aspects of primary process. Thus Needles (1959) reflected the prevailing view in stating: "Gesticulation as an accompaniment of, or substitute for, speech bears all the earmarks of regressive behavior . . . [and] represents a return to an infantile level of functioning . . . " (p. 292–293). It was from within this context that Deutsch (1947, 1952) carried out his pioneering work of relating the verbal themes of his patient's utterances to their preferred postures on the couch, devising for this purpose stick figure "posturegrams" to capture their major alignments. The beauty and authenticity of these observations was overshadowed, however, by Deutsch's efforts to elaborate a theoretical psychosomatic formulation to account for these behaviors in terms of repression and regressive deployment of libidinal energy.

In a similar vein, during a 1969 panel exploration of nonverbal communication (Suslick 1969), the power of this old constraint can still be seen, as well as the struggle to transcend it. Zeligs is noted as referring to posturing and gesturing as more primitive forms of nonverbal communication (p. 960). Rangell (1954) and Adatto (1970), both with earlier contributions made upon the significance of hand–snout kinesics in relation to poise and social–sexual anxiety, found it necessary to affirm the analytic need that such behaviors be pursued to full verbal articulation. Arlow (Suslick 1969, p. 961) provided a four-part generalization about nonverbal behaviors cast exclusively in the metaphor of the written word: nonverbal acts are a punctuation that emphasizes or modifies the verbal, are a glossary that explains or elaborates the text, or are footnoting commentary upon what is verbalized. Furthermore, they are automatisms resulting from the eruption of dissociated, highly organized mental activity. Three of these describe the nonverbal in strictly literate, verbal metaphor, and as subordinated to the latter. The fourth assigns the nonverbal to the realm of the dynamic unconscious and repressed, yet still to be compared to a palimpsest, a used parchment previously written upon.

What is striking is that Arlow went on to provide a clinically sensitive scanning of the rich significance of the nonverbal in the analysis of a never silent and gesturally busy patient who had been raised by deaf-mute parents and habitually signed as he spoke. This patient feared dumbness, even as from the beginning he had learned to communicate in the family sign language they had devised. It became necessary for the patient to translate this other language for the sake of the analyst's understanding. The latter saw this signing as motor communication alluding to parental transference.

Recognition of the full potentiality of gestural expressiveness for our psychoanalytic work has been nearly as slow in coming as has been the acknowledgment of the unique powers of natural sign language for the congenitally deaf. For their field it would take many years of practical experience and research, documented eloquently by Oliver Sacks (1989), to override the prevailing bias that the deaf should learn oral speech, and to demonstrate the natural signing of the deaf to be a complete and supple language in its own right, superior to mere words in its power of portrayal in a four-dimensional fashion.

In our field we have had an equivalent struggle to realize a comparable affirmation of the power and depth of nonverbal expression in those of us who also speak. The older emphasis on the regressive and primitive significance of the nonverbal components of human communication, traditionally viewed as synonymous with primary process, only slowly has been challenged by a developmental viewpoint that would ascribe to primary process modes a continuing importance for all aspects of human behavior throughout life (McLaughlin 1978, Noy 1969).

From this developmental perspective, the nonverbal contributions of both parties to the analytic work originate in capacities we acquired during those formative years when nonverbal interactions were the primary carriers of the infant's communicating with his mother. Action and gesture were there from the beginnings of our internal psychic life, central to its unfolding and affective enrichment. We learned to trust this level of speaking and knowing more deeply than the words that came later, and few have put aside an awareness of what gestures and body language had to tell us. In the repetition and familiarity that mark the analytic work these nonverbal contributions become recognizable, deepening the experiential and affective dimensions of the analytic exchange for both, not just as a remnant of the developmental past, but as an essential, continuing enrichment of the full range of subtlety and nuance of our words that carry the analytic dialogue.

I know that I am pleading a personal bias in claiming such importance for observational data that can carry little relevance for those analysts, and there are many, who do not need kinesic cues to inform their work. I do need and utilize this visual, multisensorial input. This is linked to my perceptual style of analytic listening. Not blessed with a strong capability for visual imagery, I make much use of my kinesthetic-affective responses in tracking and resonating to my patients. I need to look while I listen. As Mushatt put it during yet another panel discussion (Lilleskov 1977), analysts were also subject to sensory deprivation in the analytic situation, particularly when they did not attend to the patient's nonverbal behavior. It is noteworthy that by then some of the contributors seemed to accept that valid meaning could be gleaned from attending to the nonverbal and were more concerned with technical issues of how and when to deal with these communications.

By now there is a substantial literature on the matter (Anthi 1983, Jacobs 1973, McLaughlin 1987, Shapiro 1979). Jacobs (1991) in particular has described well how the analyst's own kinesic and inner bodily experiences provide valuable data alluding to the dynamic processes current in both.

My particular focus in this presentation has been on the possibility of amassing clinical data that might collectively attest to relevant linkage between persistent kinesic phenomena seen in adult patients and the developmental vicissitudes of their very early years. I put it thus because in matters like these, there is no way to make clear any linear connections. Perhaps the best that can be done is to identify similarities of theme and mode, gathered from as many aspects of the particular analytic experience as can be noted, and to allow these collectively to converge in their own fashion, to shape or mime a pattern or mosaic that might show fit or match with the past.

The two clinical instances given here involve dynamic issues that overlap and provide a complementarity to each other, both in terms of their adult behaviors in analysis and in terms of how these two patients experienced their early mothering and maturational struggles.

Mr. E., a solid obsessional with only moderate problems at the oedipal level, saw himself as caught up in larger conflicts centered on his relationship to his mother, with whom he seemed from his early days to have been in trouble. Matters of freedom, autonomy, reliable nurturance, and rapid propulsion through the times of feeding, weaning, and achieving sphincter control, all were suffused with the turmoil of casual and erratic mothering, worsened by punitive demands for compliance and obligatory attachment.

Here the similarities with Mrs. T. are evident. Although the qualities of mothering were different, insofar as Mrs. T.'s mother seemed much more available and reliably responsive to her child's physical discomforts, there is good evidence to support Mrs. T.'s perceptions of her mother as expecting a similarly docile alacrity in getting through the early acquisition of control and autonomy of body functions. Similarly, mother put much constraint upon her daughter's freedoms and autonomy at all levels of expression, using not physical coercion but induction of guilt felt in relation to a suffering mother, then a punitive god.

Both patients showed as adults much shame around adequacy of performance and uncertainty of the reality and ownership of their bodies and capacities. Both felt themselves perpetually in a dangerous struggle over claiming their accomplishments in their adult work and personal life, and earlier from a mother who seemed to need to own and control all. Both clung to regressive ways of soothing their oral hunger and rage: Mr. E. with his "I'll get it for myself" snacking, as well as his intractable nail biting; Mrs. T. with her mouthing of baubles and fingers and her resort to solitary wine drinking at night.

For both, it is possible to trace rather clear connections between these contemporary manifestations of oral dependency and their historical antecedents receding into early developmental time. Mr. E.'s accounts of battles with his mother over his nail biting and thumb sucking emerged in the analysis in accompaniment to his actual nail picking and thumb picking, plus mute evidence of renewed nail biting outside the analytic hours. Mrs. T.'s behaviors with her necklace—mouthing, clutching, hurling away—occurred as she brought out her rage and fear over concerns about me having to do with her need for nurturance and her fear of deprivation and abandonment. She went on from these to make affectively rich recounting of her forced weaning and hurried toilet training, accomplished in a context of parental censure for any oral protest.

Both patients played out kinesically their oscillating between a reach for autonomy and separateness and their need for protected closeness. Mr. E. did so very quietly in his overall stillness on the couch, with only his hands in action, his fingers and thumbs pantomiming in affirmation, at times contradiction, of his verbally expressed wishes and concerns. Mrs. T. could also be quiet in playing out these themes, as in her trinket play. She more often was dramatic in her whole-body behaviors, as in looking back to make eye contact; turning to me in abject pleading or coming at me in roaring fury, weapon in hand;

running to the glass boundary between my space and the outside world; or hovering on the threshold, either to return to the couch as a submissive heap or bolt through the door and be gone. Her stirrup ritual, though from a later time, also portrayed this conflict in graphic tensional poignancy, as she literally immobilized herself in a position of vulnerability by preventing her feet from flying.

Winnicott's (1953) concept of transitional phenomena and objects comes into focus as a construct overlapping those of separation and rapprochement. I think that some of Mr. E.'s gentler finger and thumb kinesics can be viewed as a carryover of transitional usages. The justification lies in the clear-enough temporal linkage between these behaviors and the verbal content speaking his needs for soothing and sheltering from wife or from me, along with his recalling how he did turn to and receive some affection and caring from his sister in his toddler years. I think of an attenuation, a kind of wistful reminiscence, in such small kinesics that alludes to once-important, early dynamic issues now revived in the multiple layering of the analytic transference. In Mr. E.'s case, the allusion would be to a time when a very small boy found in his thumb sucking such transitional aid and solace by which to handle his need for more nurturance and comfort.

In Mrs. T.'s instance, I had the impression that her ways of using her necklace and bodice, to grasp and fondle, then violently throw aside, put into action her uncertain grasp of the comfort of a transitional object. These behaviors, repeated over and over, seemed in consonance with, and part of her shaky grasp on, object constancy, so very prominent in her relationship to me.

I find another level of confirmatory evidence in the relationship vicissitudes of enactment and tension that my patients and I fell into, tested and found helpful or hindering, as we struggled to make headway in the work. I feel that the data I have provided point to high intensities of anxiety and regression in both patients in response to my behaviors that struck them as threatening their autonomy and boundaries, even as they simultaneously hungered for my solace and rescue. Both needed, and responded quite positively yet differently to, behaviors of mine that acknowledged their right to own what they clung to as their own, and allowed them gradually to be both close to and apart from me with less turmoil. At such times either patient could allow me a freer field in which to contribute my own reflective metaphor, cued by the metaphor of their nonverbal behaviors. Together we often came upon levels of highly charged transference actualization, leading to affectively rich recollection of the troubled past.

As I conclude I know that all I have been able to gather about separation–attachment issues from my clinical data from adult analyses must be acknowledged to be a collage of circumstantial evidence. I would hope these are sufficient to support my general view of the effective psychoanalytic experience as a prolonged enactment or actualization in which nonverbal behaviors have an essential role. I have tried to fashion a dramatic unity out of the words of patient and analyst, along with their large and small actions, that portray the themes of past and present. Through transference these come alive in the mind of the patient and analyst and are enacted between the pair in the analytic moment; they then blend in the music of the affective experiences of both parties to authenticate the whole.

Sacks (1989) has described how readily even the hearing inhabitants of Martha's Vineyard tended to resort to the natural signing of their community. "They would slip into it, involuntarily, sometimes in the middle of a sentence, because Sign is 'natural' to all who learn it (as a primary language), and has an intrinsic beauty and excellence sometimes superior to speech" (p. 35).

I would like to extend Sacks's observation to include all of us, even though we are certainly not sign-fluent, so as to remind us of what we know: that we constantly provide stamp and signature for what we are, and for what we feel, through our posture, gestures, facial expressions, voice qualities, and the rest. That to a varying extent we are forever signers, as well as speakers, because we spent so many years in rapt mimetic absorption of our world, before we had words to supplement these alternative ways of knowing and telling. And that we do not lose or relinquish these ways just because there are times when words are better.

REFERENCES

Adatto, C. (1970). Snout-hand behavior in an adult patient. *Journal of the American Psychoanalytic Association* 18:823-830.
Anthi, P. (1983). Reconstruction of preverbal experiences. *Journal of the American Psychoanalytic Association* 31:33-59.
Deutsch, F. (1947). Analysis of postural behaviors. *Psychoanalytic Quarterly* 16:195-213.
——— (1952). Analytic posturology. *Psychoanalytic Quarterly* 21:196-214.
Eissler, K. (1953). The effect of the structure of the ego on psychoanalytic technique. *Journal of the American Psychoanalytic Association* 1:104-143.
——— (1958). Remarks on some variations in psychoanalytic technique. *International Journal of Psycho-Analysis* 39:222-229.
Ferenczi, S. (1919). Thinking and muscle Innervation. In *Further Contributions to the Theory and Technique of Psychoanalysis,* pp. 230-232. New York: Basic Books, 1952.
Freud, S. (1905). Three essays on the theory of sexuality. *Standard Edition* 7:135-243.
——— (1911). The dynamics of transference. *Standard Edition* 12:97-108.
——— (1912). Recommendations to physicians practising psycho-analysis. *Standard Edition* 12:109-120.
——— (1913). On beginning the treatment (further recommendations on the technique of psycho-analysis I). *Standard Edition* 12:123-144.
——— (1914). Remembering, repeating and working-through (further recommendations on the technique of psycho-analysis II). *Standard Edition* 12:144-156.
——— (1923). The ego and the id. *Standard Edition* 19:3-66.
Groddeck, G. (1928). *The Book of It.* New York: Nervous and Mental Disease Publishing.
Horowitz, M. (1978). *Image Formation and Cognition.* New York: Appleton-Century-Crofts.
Jacobs, T. (1973). Posture, gesture and movement in the analyst: cues to interpretation and countertransference. *Journal of the American Psychoanalytic Association* 21:77-92.

——— (1991). *The Use of the Self.* Madison, CT: International Universities Press.
Kramer, S. (1979). The technical significance and application of Mahler's separation-individuation theory. *Journal of the American Psychoanalytic Association* 27:207-240.
Lilleskov, R. (1977). Nonverbal aspects of child and adult psychoanalysis. *Journal of the American Psychoanalytic Association* 25:679-692.
Mahler, M., Pine, F., and Bergman, A. (1975). *The Psychological Birth of the Human Infant.* New York: Basic Books.
McLaughlin, J. (1978). Primary and secondary process in the context of cerebral hemispheric specialization. *Psychoanalytic Quarterly* 47:237-266.
——— (1987). The play of transference: some reflections on enactment in the psychoanalytic situation. *Journal of the American Psychoanalytic Association* 35:557-582.
Needles, W. (1959). Gesticulation and speech. *International Journal of Psycho-Analysis* 40:291-294.
Noy, P. (1969). A revision of the psychoanalytic theory of the primary process. *International Journal of Psycho-Analysis* 50:155-178.
Rangell, L. (1954). The psychology of poise: psychic significance of the snout. *International Journal of Psycho-Analysis* 35:313-332.
Sacks, O. (1989). *Seeing Voices: A Journey into the World of the Deaf.* Berkeley, CA: University of California Press.
Shapiro, T. (1979). *Clinical Psycholinguistics.* New York: Plenum.
Suslick, A. (1969). Nonverbal communication in the analysis of adults. *Journal of the American Psychoanalytic Association* 17:955-967.
Winnicott, D. (1953). Transitional objects and transitional phenomena. *International Journal of Psycho-Analysis* 34:89-97.

7

GESTURES, EMBLEMS, AND BODY LANGUAGE: WHAT DOES IT ALL MEAN?

Discussion of McLaughlin's Chapter: "Nonverbal Behaviors in the Analytic Situation: The Search for Meaning in Nonverbal Cues"

Sydney E. Pulver, M.D.

As we have come to expect, Dr. James T. McLaughlin has given us a superb account of his topic, nonverbal communication and the meaning of the patient's behavior on the couch. I realize that discussions such as this are best when they are critical, but I cannot begin the critique without pointing out the virtues of this presentation. McLaughlin writes eloquently, in a lyrical style that not only captures and conveys the dynamics of his patients, but also provides a description of the interaction between patient and analysand in a way that is rare in our literature. His theoretical and technical accomplishments are evident. He conveys his theory unobtrusively yet convincingly, and his psychoanalytic technique emerges without the idealization of the analyst that so many of our writers convey. He emerges from these pages as a gentle yet firm man, an analyst who knows what he is doing and is sure enough of himself to be able to state his uncertainties ("I was wrong in my assumption . . ."; "I was first surprised and a bit abashed . . ."; "I felt some anxious press to reclaim the right to speak for myself . . .") without being defensive about them.

The sense of competency that McLaughlin conveys is due in no small part to his unalloyed conviction that analysis is a therapy that takes place in a relationship in which each participant is constantly shaping and being shaped by the other. It may be true that the analyst is somewhat less malleable than the analysand. However, no good analyst escapes being strongly influenced in both feelings and view of reality by his analysand. Nor does he escape from doing such influencing himself, despite his most valiant efforts to the contrary. McLaughlin is a social constructivist (Hoffman 1991) and was one long before that view of the analytic process became fashionable. A central tenet of this position is that what used to be thought of only as transference–countertransference enactments are a ubiquitous and invariable part of the mutual interaction in every analysis. Understanding them is a crucial part of the analytic process. McLaughlin (1987) has pointed out elsewhere that what are usually called manifestations of transference are frequently transference–countertransference enactments of this sort and need to be analyzed as such. Such enactments are not only unavoidable in any analysis in which the analyst is optimally involved with the patient, but are desirable in that their analysis almost always moves the analysis forward (Schwaber 1990). McLaughlin's recognition of this is demonstrated in such passages as his description of an interaction with Mrs. T.: "These breakdowns [of rapport] between us often were triggered by certain behaviors of mine as I tried to meet and understand her quicksilver challenges and pleas for rescue or guidance."

KINESICS AND ENACTMENTS

A major thrust of this chapter is to point out the particular value of kinesics in detecting transference–countertransference enactments. We often note them not only by the verbal responses of the patient or by the perceptions our own feelings but, just as important, by the nonverbal responses to which McLaughlin is calling our attention. A patient of mine had been describing at some length some egregiously nasty behavior of her mother, behavior that we were coming to see was illustrative of her mother's self-centeredness, critical nature, and inability to empathize with the patient's feelings and wishes. After her description of one incident that had particularly upset her, I asked her how she felt her mother had been feeling when she acted as she did. She tried to address this question, but there was a peculiar distance and deadness in her response. Her hands, previously gesticulating, were silent. Her entire upper torso, previously animatedly engaged in the description, now lay still on the couch, and there was a flattening in the tone of her voice. I commented on the change and asked whether it was connected with my question. After a little thought, she realized that my question had led her to feel that I hadn't been with her during the entire session. She was interested in conveying to me the agony she felt when her mother was being outrageous, while I seemed to be more interested in her mother. Furthermore, there was a hint of criticism in the way I asked the question, as if I were saying, "Stop feeling so sorry for yourself and pay a little attention to your mother." And, I came to realize, I was to some degree doing just that. My overt intent had been to help the patient deal with her mother's behavior by understanding some of the feelings that were behind it. Without realizing it, however, I had become impatient with my patient's litany of complaints and was covertly telling her to shape up and be constructive. As she and I explored what had happened between us, she made the first step in a gradually dawning understanding of a pervasive process. The same thing that happened between the two of us often happened between her and her mother. Her mother's hostile behavior arose not just from her own hostility, but because my patient provoked her to irritation and criticism. This opened new vistas toward an understanding of my patient's intricate relationship with her mother. It is typical of the way that an exploration of transference–countertransference enactments can be fruitful.

Other aspects of McLaughlin's technique are worth commenting upon. In his work with Mrs. T. he demonstrates elegantly the way in which we gradually find out what is best for our patients. At the beginning of therapy, we are two individuals getting to know each other. In carrying out the mutual task of coming to understand the patient, the analyst is manifestly interested in him. The patient is less openly but just as eagerly interested in the analyst. Our interventions, whether interpretations or modes of reacting in various situations, are tentative. We do what needs to be done to keep the analytic situation going, but we learn what that is only imperfectly and gradually. Luckily, our patients are tolerant and our mistakes fruitful, if only we recognize them and try to understand them with the patient. The description of this process of mutual groping toward insight is often poorly conveyed in our case reports. McLaughlin sets it forth in a way that enables every analyst to recognize his own experience.

McLaughlin's point is that our patients convey a great deal to us about themselves beyond the information that is carried in the words they say. Communication takes place on many levels, and the nonverbal levels are as important, and often more important, than the verbal ones. As in our work with words, we do not leap to conclusions. This precept was brought home to me a few days after I had accepted the assignment of discussing McLaughlin's chapter. My interest in my patients' nonverbal behavior was at a peak. I was relatively successful in understanding most of it, so I was particularly intrigued when I could not understand the peculiar arm motions of a young man in analysis. He seemed to alternate between two positions on the couch. Much of the time he would lie with upper arms on the couch and his hands clasped together on his chest in what appeared to be a benign and tranquil attitude. However, from time to time he would fold his arms together tightly in what I had always taken in other patients to be a gesture of willful defiance. The problem was that at these times he did not seem to be defiant in any other way, verbally or nonverbally. I carefully tracked these alternations of arm position and for several weeks was unable to make any dynamic sense of them. One day, however, at a moment when I was not consciously puzzling over the phenomenon, realization struck. He would fold his arms tightly across his chest every time the compressor on my air conditioner cycled on! Thankfully, I had refrained from pointing out this significant behavior, and I gained a slightly wider perspective about the possible meanings of nonverbal behavior.

McLaughlin traces the psychoanalytic history of nonverbal communication. I would like to supplement that by looking at the history of such understanding in general psychology. As so often happens, analytic understanding and progress in general psychology often develop simultaneously, but with little reference to each other. In this case, as we shall see, the psychologists were studying the more manifest meanings of nonverbal communication at the same time that McLaughlin and other psychoanalysts (Deutsch 1947, Freud 1915, Groddeck 1928) were focusing on the latent content. Incidentally, nonverbal communication is a designation that embraces not only the phenomena McLaughlin is describing in his chapter, but also many other modes of communication out of the verbal realm and only incidentally connected to body motion. More about that later.

McLaughlin mentions kinesics, the name given to the study of bodily motion by one of the outstanding investigators of the area in recent times, Ray Birdwhistell (1970). As Birdwhistell points out, the fact that formalized gestures play a role in communication has been known almost from time immemorial. In the first half of the twentieth century, that role had captured the interest of numerous investigators (Allport and Vernon 1933, Dunlap 1927, James 1932, Krout 1931, Wolff 1945), but the actual theory and methodology of "expressive communication" were not developed until the earlier work of Birdwhistell (1952) and Scheflen (1963). The latter hoped to develop "a methodology, an annotational system, and a set of norms," that is, a science, kinesiology, instead of kinesics. While to a large extent they succeeded, the term "kinesiology" never gained acceptance. The study of communication by bodily motion was gradually merged into the broader field of nonverbal communication. This field drew a great deal of interest in the early 1970s, a development that can be followed in the index entries in *Psychological Abstracts*. Until 1969, kinesics appeared only sporadically under the heading of "Communication non-verbal." In 1971, this became "Communication, Non-Verbal," and in 1973 "Non-Verbal Communication," a heading it has maintained until the present. "Kinesics," when it appears, is indexed on the same level as such other entries as gestures, smile, and body language.

MODES OF NONVERBAL BEHAVIOR

McLaughlin originally subtitled his chapter "The Search for Meaning in Kinetic Cues." The current title, in which "nonverbal" is substituted for "kinetic," reflects his recognition that kinetic cues are only one kind of nonverbal behavior. It seems to me that the various modes of nonverbal behavior, and their communicative implications, have not been thoroughly studied and diagrammed. Their origins and meaning in particular are understood only in a rather helter-skelter way. If we are to carry McLaughlin's work further, we must distinguish between gestures, which are a main focus of his interest, and other types of nonverbal communication. We must also have some idea of the origins and different meanings of the various types of gestures, and some inkling about how they relate to other nonverbal communications. To help clarify this, I will attempt a rough categorization of nonverbal behaviors, with particular emphasis on hand movements.

Bodily movements, as I mentioned, are only one kind of

nonverbal communication. Among the others are facial expression; posture (overall, in contrast to specific bodily movements); autonomic nervous system manifestations such as sweating, tachycardia, blanching, and tachypnea; style and manner of talking; and tone of voice. McLaughlin focuses mainly on bodily movements, a complex topic. To appreciate this complexity, consider the various kinds of body movements that can be delineated: intentional acts, manifestations of posture, arm, leg, and body movements that are expressions of affect (e.g., foot tapping and finger drumming), and gestures. The latter consisted of two distinct forms, emblems and gestures proper. Emblems are "gestures that have a specific social code of their own, have conventional paraphrases or names, are learned as separate symbols, and can be used as if they were spoken words..." (McNeill 1985, p. 351). In some cases, emblems are systematically spelled out, as in American Sign Language. In others, they are part of a culture's communication technique, known to everyone but not usually formally described or systematized. When I wish to tell a friend that I have doubts about the sanity of a colleague and do so by tapping my head with my forefinger, I am using an emblem. Some cultures, such as Italian, make extensive use of emblems; others, such as English, relatively little. Emblems differ from gestures in that they are interpretable in the absence of speech, while gestures are not. We might define gestures as "movements that ... occur only during speech, are synchronized with linguistic units, [and] are parallel in semantic and pragmatic function to the synchronized linguistic units..." (p. 351). Cognitive psychology is at present engaged in a debate about gestures. Much of McLaughlin's chapter deals with gestures. His main point is that a study of these gestures in the psychoanalytic situation contributes greatly to our understanding of our patients. This is undoubtedly true. Since it would seem that such a study might also contribute in a significant way to the aforementioned debate, let us look at it in a little more detail.

The debate is summarized by two recent articles: McNeill

(1985) and Feyereisen (1987). McNeill argues that "gestures and speech are parts of the same psychological structure and share a computational stage" (p. 350). By this he means that, after one formulates an idea that one wishes to convey, a process of linguistic computations takes place as one gets ready to speak. A "covert verbal plan" is developed, and from this plan are generated both verbal utterances (speech) and gestures. Both speech and gestures express either the same or different aspects of the covert verbal plan, arise concurrently as aspects of a single expressive structure, and can thus be said to share the same computational stage. Feyereisen argues to the contrary. Among the many pieces of evidence that McNeill marshals to support his thesis is that gestures have parallel semantic and pragmatic functions. That is, gestures and concurrent speech always express aspects of the same underlying concept, the particular concept the speaker is attempting to communicate. It is here that McLaughlin's observations, and those of other psychoanalysts, seem to provide both supportive and contradictory evidence. Mrs. T.'s behavior with her necklace (the mouthing, clutching, and hurling away) seem very likely to be manifestations of a need for nurturance and fear of deprivation and abandonment, as McLaughlin describes. In the material he presents, they occur at the same time that Mrs. T. is putting those feelings into words in her interactions with him. Analysts, however, tend to be interested in latent content. The gestures that analysts are interested in are those that are *not* expressive of the verbal ideas being conveyed by the patient. These are illustrated by Mr. E.'s "comforting" hand movements, which, while at times were correlated with overt speech about the need for comforting or reassurance from his wife, at other times were indicative of this need *while he was overtly speaking of something else.*

A more dramatic example of this was given me by Dr. David Walzer. A young woman whom he was seeing in analysis began, when she became anxious on the couch, what at first looked like the typical handwringing that occurs in anxiety.

During the analysis, however, it became clear that this hand-wringing was really a hand restraining, and that it represented an attempt to defend against a desire to masturbate with which she struggled when she was feeling sexually aroused in the transference and was anxious about it. At these times the actual verbal material was frequently related to anxious sexual yearnings, but it sometimes would deal with things that were entirely unrelated and that were being talked about as a defense against the sexual ideas. It would seem in cases like this that, while there is a link between the words and the gestures, the link occurs a significant distance prior to the formulation of the covert verbal plan, and the language and the gestures do not share the same computational stage. One could argue that these gestures are a different phenomenon than the gestures McNeill is speaking about. If so, at the very least a new definition of gestures is needed. Perhaps hand movements that occur during speech, are synchronized with linguistic units, and perform text functions like speech should only be considered gestures if they are parallel in semantic and pragmatic function. My own sense is that this is probably true, and that the gestures that share the same computational stage are different from the gestures that arise at other times in the expression of underlying feelings and ideas. Just what we would call those gesturelike movements that are not correlated directly with the covert verbal plan can be left to future students of the subject. We need, of course, not only a different name for them, but a more detailed study of all of their characteristics.

We have, then, a variety of nonverbal behaviors involving the hands. First, we have gestures in their most commonly used sense: hand movements that accompany speech, deal with the same ideas being expressed manifestly, and seem to arise from the same computational platform. Second, there are those very similar movements that express ideas and feelings that are active in the individual's thinking but are not being expressed verbally at the moment, and, we infer, are not being thought about consciously. Third, we have "emblems," stylized culturally determined hand movements with specific meanings of their own. Finally, there are the hand movements that are expressions of inhibited affective states, such as finger drumming in anxiety or impatience. All in all, hand movements are a complex phenomenon, worthy of much more detailed psychoanalytic investigation, for which McLaughlin's work provides an auspicious beginning.

Turning now to some other aspects of McLaughlin's discussion, let me first address the question he raises of whether the phenomena he describes are in fact manifestations of separation–individuation. My reaction is mixed. Mahler (1968) described the separation–individuation process as a comprehensive one including its forerunners, the normal autistic phase and the normal symbiotic phase. The separation–individuation phase proper begins at the height of symbiosis, around age 5 to 6 months, and continues at least until 24 months. Certainly much of the material McLaughlin describes is related to problems that occur in the first two years of life, and the separation–individuation process goes on at least during that developmental period. But separation–individuation is a specific process involving the separation from mother and the formation of the sense of the self as an individual. It does *not* refer to all aspects of the relationship with mother, nor does it refer to all aspects of the development of a sense of self. Generalizing the meaning of separation–individuation to all relationships with objects and all aspects of the developing self renders the term meaningless. Furthermore, as Pine (1979) pointed out, phenomena in adults that have the manifest appearance of phenomena occurring in separation–individuation are not necessarily linearly related to that phase. In fact, they are often distant derivatives originating ultimately in the separation–individuation phase but having gone through great modifications in subsequent development. Looking at McLaughlin's clinical data in the narrower and more specific sense of the term, I suspect that much of the nonverbal behavior he describes, early though it is, does not relate specifically to separation–individuation. At least, the evidence for such a relationship is unclear.

TECHNICAL IMPLICATIONS

Next, let us consider the clinical utility of these phenomena. Analyzing nonverbal behavior requires considerable finesse. In his 1987 article, McLaughlin differentiated between the obvious ("those behaviors which strike the eye as unusual and idiosyncratic") and the more subtle ("the more ubiquitous, unobtrusive behaviors that generally go unnoticed"). Analyzing the latter is much more difficult than the former. A comparison to the analysis of character traits might be helpful in understanding this. "Analyzing," of course, describes the process in which the patient and the analyst gain a joint understanding of some aspect of the patient's behavior in a way that the patient can use to modify that behavior if he so desires. Analysts often understand, to a more or less deep degree, some aspect of their patient's behavior, but we do not say that the behavior is analyzed until the patient also understands it and can utilize that understanding. For the patient to cooperate with the analyst in this endeavor, he must first recognize that the behavior in question exists as something that is patterned and repetitive. He must then *desire* to understand the behavior. It must, that is, become ego dystonic. This is standard practice in analyzing character traits and would appear to be true also for nonverbal behavior. If an analyst notes (perhaps in the transference) that a patient characteristically makes sarcastic comments about the appearance of others (a character trait), his first step in analyzing this is to help the patient become aware that he is engaging in it. This often requires a great deal of time and tact, since most character traits are not only ego syntonic but feel like a part of the self and serve important defensive purposes. Once the patient is aware of it, he must then come to see that the character trait is less serviceable, or at least less innocuous than it had been felt to be. Only then will the patient become interested in exploring and changing it. From the standpoint of analyzing, nonverbal behavior functions exactly the same as character traits. First, the patient must become aware of the behavior, something that is much easier to accomplish when the behavior is unusual and idiosyncratic than when it is subtle. Next, the patient must be motivated to understand what the behavior represents. For this to happen, he must become convinced that in fact there is some significance to what he is doing and that it is deleterious to him. This kind of awareness and conviction is easier to arrive at when the behavior is obtrusive than when it is natural and subtle. My experience agrees with McLaughlin's. It is rarely useful to call a patient's attention directly to any kind of nonverbal behavior, whether subtle or obvious, either by inquiring about it directly (I notice that you always keep one foot on the floor while you lie on the couch. Do you have any thoughts about that?) or by interpreting it in isolation as the initial approach to a conflict (I wonder if you keep one foot on the floor to reassure yourself that you can leave whenever you want to.) Patients often react to such attempts with bemused acceptance and polite inquisitiveness, but this is usually nonproductive; the nonverbal behavior often disappears from the scene. One is most likely to effectively utilize nonverbal behaviors in interpretation when they can be linked with an overall understanding of the patient's behavior. When it becomes clear or almost clear to the patient that he indeed wants to be free to leave, linking the one foot on the floor with the various other precautions he takes to be sure of his freedom can be very productive. In brief, nonverbal behaviors are most useful clinically to help the analyst in understanding. Occasionally, however, when they are specific and idiosyncratic they can lead to an exploration of an unconscious conflict, usually connected with a traumatic event.

CONCLUSION

In closing, let me reiterate that McLaughlin has made an important contribution to the understanding of nonverbal behavior in the analytic situation. In our present age of social constructivism, the role of nonverbal behavior in understanding the interactions between analyst and patient is bound to grow increasingly important. Analysts will need to pay more attention to the affective status of the patient and the impact of traumatic events, both of which are exquisitely revealed in the nonverbal sphere. Finally, as I have tried to show, the implications of McLaughlin's studies extend beyond analysis and will have important bearing upon the work of other students of human behavior.

REFERENCES

Allport, G. W., and Vernon, P. E. (1933). *Studies in Expressive Movements.* New York: Macmillan.

Birdwhistell, R. L. (1952). *Introduction to Kinesics.* Louisville, KY: University of Louisville Press.

——— (1970). *Kinesics and Content: Essays on Body Motion Communication.* Philadelphia: University of Pennsylvania Press.

Deutsch, F. (1947). Analysis of postural behavior. *Psychoanalytic Quarterly* 16:195–213.

Dunlap, K. (1927). A project for investigating the facial signs of personality. *Journal of Psychology* 39:156–161.

Feyereisen, P. (1987). Gestures and speech, interactions and separations. *Psychological Review* 94:493–498.

Freud, S. (1915). Introductory lectures on psycho-analysis. *Standard Edition* 15:15–79.

Groddeck, G. (1923). *The Book of It.* New York: Nervous and Mental Disease Publishing.

Hoffman, I. Z. (1991). Discussion: toward a social-constructivist view of the psychoanalytic situation. *Psychoanalytic Dialogues* 1:74–125.

James, W. T. (1932). A study of the expression of bodily posture. *Journal of Genetic Psychology* 7:405–437.

Krout, M. H. (1931). Symbolic gestures in the clinical study of personality. *Transactions of Illinois State Academy of Science* 24:519–523.

Mahler, S. (1968). *On Human Symbiosis and the Vicissitudes of Individuation.* New York: International Universities Press.

McLaughlin, J. T. (1987). The play of transference: some reflections on enactment in the psychoanalytic situation. *Journal of the American Psychoanalytic Association* 35:557–582.

McNeill, D. (1985). So you think gestures are nonverbal? *Psychological Review* 92:350–371.

Pine, F. (1979). On the pathology of the separation–individuation process as manifested in later clinical work: an attempt at delineation. *International Journal of Psycho-Analysis* 60:225–242.

Scheflen, A. E. (1963). Aims and methods in psychotherapy. In *Psychosomatic Medicine*, ed. J. H. Nodine and J. H. Moyer, pp. 748–752. Philadelphia: Lea and Febiger.

Schwaber, E. (1990). Interpretation and the therapeutic action of psychoanalysis. *International Journal of Psycho-Analysis* 71:229–240.

Wolff, C. (1945). *Psychology of Gesture*. London: Methuen.

8

TECHNICAL APPLICATIONS OF THE NONVERBAL ASPECTS OF SEPARATION-INDIVIDUATION PHENOMENA

A Concluding Commentary on Akhtar's, Frank's, and McLaughlin's Chapters

Bernard L. Pacella, M.D.

A most difficult task confronting the contemporary psychoanalyst is the valid application and integration of the data from early child development research, especially the observations of Mahler and colleagues (1975), into psychoanalytic theory and practice. Their work suggests that a connection may exist between a current manifest behavior in an adult and a specific type of behavior during the separation–individuation phase of development. For instance, if during the practicing phase (approximately ages 10 to 16 months), a child is allowed considerable freedom in activity with very little restraint by both parents and is kissed and hugged excessively over any slight performance, and this overwhelming indulgence is maintained throughout adolescence, there may be such tremendous fostering of the developing sense of omnipotence as to stimulate excessive preoccupations and actions that are in the service of this omnipotence and at the same time interfere with the development of the reality-testing function. Could this foster the development of "personal myths" (Kris 1956) and generate "derivative" patterns of behavior throughout the later years, which can be recognized in the course of analytic work?

THE DEVELOPMENTAL BACKDROP

Certainly, in Mahler and colleagues' (1975) descriptions of the separation–individuation process, certain patterns of behavior during the first few years of life are correlated with specific parental attitudes toward the child. These behavioral actions and reactions of the children may be transformed or enhanced through the subsequent action of repression and other defense mechanisms as well as by the internalization processes in association with the impact of environmental factors. Yet, despite an unending series of internal and external events, specific "core patterns" (not necessarily related to the "basic core" of Weil 1970) may remain sufficiently constant as to maintain these behavior patterns, so that they are readily discernible as "derivative" patterns in the adult, modified, of course, by age-level appropriateness. I am suggesting also that these "core patterns" have the ability to act as "core magnets," which in the course of development actively seek out and screen external stimuli in order to either discard or accept appropriate stimuli for its own purposes. I have elsewhere hypothesized that

> a waking screen exists as a function of the primal matrix configuration corresponding with Lewin's concept of the dream screen. It consists of a primitive parental configuration referable to the symbiotic and the separation–individuation periods of life as a kind of basic memory complex acting as an organizing function of the ego. It exerts its influence in varying degrees upon the dynamic-economic aspects of psychic activity. The earliest sensory experience with the symbiotic mother and later experiences with the parents during the separation–individuation process form the early matrix which continues to act as a "waking screen." The matrix memory complex represents the anchor

upon which new objects and new experiences impinge. It plays an active role in scanning, integrating, rejecting or modifying all the newer percepts of object representations throughout life. It is a specifically woven fabric derived from the primitive ego representing a basic core from which further objects relations develop, and toward which regressive or return paths allow for rapid retreat to the safety of reunion with the primal love object. [Pacella 1980, pp. 129–130]

In the course of development, the principles of optimum or maximum familiarity and safety (Sandler 1960) operate and permit the infant and child to add to the core patterns those new inputs that would be familiar, pleasurable, or economically acceptable. This early patterning would be more attractive to the "infant system" early in life and therefore more in the service of the pleasure-pain principle, thus more attuned to the representations of the care-giving or mother representation. As the child begins to crawl and move away from the mother, thereby enlarging its orbit or sphere of activity wherein the mother is still in view, it must adapt to other external objects and surroundings that must be added on to the maternal representations of its original world. At this point, the adaptive and safety principles come into play, and an increasingly complex series of incorporative developments occur as cognitive function and memory develop. The infant broadens its involvement with the external milieu and other objects during the practicing subphase of separation–individuation, while at the same time checking to see that the mother is not far off. The child's narcissistic interests, closely intertwined with its sense of omnipotence, are badly bruised during the rapprochement subphase, when ambitendencies (perhaps the precursor of ambivalence and splitting of object representations) are gradually worked through and the core object representations become more firmly internalized, leading to the development of object constancy. With increasing structuralization of ego functions and capacities, in addition to primitive forerunners of superego development, the young child is prepared for the onset of the oedipal phase of development. Subsequent phases of life, such as adolescence and early adulthood, impact upon the early mental structures and modify them in varying degrees, depending upon a multiplicity of internal and external factors. An important question now confronts us: To what extent can these behavioral manifestations of separation–individuation be recognized in derivative forms during the later phases of life, particularly during adulthood?

It is this particular question that, in effect, is addressed by the three main contributors to this volume. They present clinical material from adult patients in psychoanalytic treatment that they feel is suggestive of remnants of the separation–individuation phase of life. This material was for them a "window" that allowed a clear view of a segment of the early dynamics between parents and the child, particularly during the rapprochement subphase of the separation–individuation process. Dr. Salman Akhtar, in his scholarly presentation, however, chooses to develop a very fascinating hypothesis of the vicissitudes of early attachment to the love object by invoking the concept of a fundamental "tether," which exerts its influence throughout life and which can be seen in its multiple manifestations in the individual. He also applies the tether idea in a multiplicity of ways to society and culture.

The three main chapters contained in this book are remarkable in their careful attention to detail and to incidental fact. They are impressive in their use of inductive logic, assessing the application of clinical material to the early life of the patient, while employing with careful strategy, deductive logic in its application to the phenomenology of separation–individuation and in developing their thesis of derivative phenomena. It is the expressed hope of the authors that they were dealing with the derivative manifestations of early behaviors and dynamic object relations, rather than pure metaphor, or merely present behavior interpreted as somewhat similar coincidental patterns. At this point, I should like to reflect more specifically on each author's contributions.

DR. AKHTAR'S CHAPTER

I must admit to being very pleasantly overwhelmed by Dr. Akhtar's chapter. Reading it was an experience of a psychoanalytic *Alice in Wonderland,* which I enjoyed immensely. At the outset, Dr. Akhtar formulates his task: "to extrapolate the ordinary English language definition of 'distance' to psychoanalytic theory," and to establish a conceptual psychodynamic order in such words as "optimal distance," distance between self and object, or two psychic structures.

He initially refers to an interesting article by Bouvet (1958) in which the "distance" taken by a patient from his analyst tends to diminish over a period of time, with variations, finally dwindling to a zero point, which Bouvet calls the "rapprocher." In effect, I believe that there is a strong element of adaptation to the "psychoanalytic situation" by the patient. A distant analogy would be a Darwinian adaptation, when, for example, an animal like the white polar bear takes on the color of snow and ice, perhaps over eons of time, as an adaptive function. The psychoanalytic "metaphor" may be the concept of mimicry and internalization of the object representation so that the subject and object now function as one person, or we might say a fusion of ego boundaries has occurred. So often the candidate in psychoanalysis takes on the gestures, language, and other forms of identity with his analyst, resembling the polar bear analogy to the environment. Would this be a lessening of distance? If so, then the process of imitating, identifying with, and internalizing all may be considered as being in the service of "rapprocher," and attaining zero distance. I am afraid this requires more thought.

I believe that Dr. Akhtar found a perfect solution regarding a useful concept of distance. Rather than restricting its definition to either intrapsychic (internal) or interpersonal (external) referents, he thought it best to accept the paradoxical way in which it is defined. He therefore acknowledges a "dialectical tension between two perspectives as being inherent to the phenomena involved," a theoretical position with which I agree thoroughly. I think it is generally agreed that to be an analyst, one must be tolerant not only of ambiguity but also of paradox. And I also agree with Dr. Akhtar that it is preferable to avoid quantifying the psychoanalytic concept of distance, since this invokes disputed aspects of the economic principle of metapsychology (i.e., quantities of psychological energy) and merely adds more ambiguity.

Dr. Akhtar discusses the concepts of Balint's (1959) proposal of two fundamental attitudes about distance from objects: the "ocnophilic" (hesitant, clinging) and the "philobatic" (thrill-loving). Dr. Akhtar then very ingeniously relates it to Spitz's (1965) observations concerning the development of visual distance perception in the infant, and additionally to Mahler and colleagues' (1975) concepts of early separation and ego boundary formation. I cannot sustain an enthusiastic position concerning the usefulness of Balint's ideas, since I am not sure as to the "purity" of the two "fundamental attitudes," but this by no means detracts from the attempt by Dr. Akhtar to reconcile different philosophic speculations and scientific observations regarding the concept of "distance," especially when he "hears" echoes in Balint's work of Mahler's recognition of "man's external struggle against both fusion and isolation" (Mahler 1972, p. 130).

Dr. Akhtar presents an excellent short summary of separation–individuation and on the basis of Mahler's observations concludes that the term "optimal distance" signifies "a psychic position which permits intimacy without loss of autonomy, and separateness without painful aloneness." This is clearly the position of Mahler, which he reiterates: "If the mother is not optimally available during the rapprochement subphase, self and object constancy is not attained, contradictory self and object representations remain split, infantile omnipotence is not renunciated, and capacity for optimal distance fails to develop. This leads to a lifelong tendency towards oscillations between passionate intimacy and hateful withdrawal from objects."

After having wrestled with a definition of "distance" and "optimal distance," Dr. Akhtar treats us to varieties of psychopathological phenomena in patients in addition to cultural phenomena involving concepts of distance, optimal distance, tethers, orbits, and invisible fences. Dr. Akhtar provides us with exceedingly relevant examples of distance, boundary, and tether phenomena in patients, in everyday life, and in social customs.

DR. FRANK'S CHAPTER

The chapter by Dr. Alvin Frank describes a case of a woman in analysis for four and a half years. It is a tale of failed developmental achievement and how it was manifested and ameliorated analytically. Prior to his case presentation, Dr. Frank, in his usual scholarly manner, provides an excellent review of other articles dealing with "couch issues." Following Freud's early comments concerning patients' dislike for lying on the couch as being in the service of resistance, subsequent reports were more substantive in dealing with the various meanings that lying on the couch has for different patients. Such meanings included an "emptiness of space"; a sense of loneliness or aloneness; a sense of humiliation or subjugation; a feeling of danger, vulnerability, and helplessness; a fear of sexual assault from the analyst; a fear of loss of sexual controls; and other concerns regarding the loss of visual contact. However, Dr. Frank mentions three references in the literature that suggest a lack of developmental capacities in certain cases where the patients cannot tolerate the "regression" (e.g., altered states of consciousness, phobic reactions) implicit in lying on the couch and thus having no visual contact with the analyst. In this connection, Dr. Frank quotes Winnicott's (1958) idea of a developmental deficit equivalent to a lack of "the capacity to be alone." This is a very significant point, and I would like to refer to at least four significant periods during the course of the separation–individuation process when the "separation from mother" issue becomes strikingly apparent:

1. During the latter half of the first year of life, and extending into the early part of the second year, when the child experiences "stranger anxiety." The child wants to hold on to or be close to his mother when a stranger appears; he may cry and avoid looking at the stranger.
2. During the "anaclitic depression" period described by Spitz (1965) for infants between the ages of 7 and 11 months. If the mother is not present, the infant may refuse the bottle and any food, lose weight, have diarrhea, vomit, and cry almost incessantly.
3. During the practicing subphase, when the child finds it necessary to keep mother always in view, or checks back visually to assure that she is still near him, even if the child wanders about as he explores.
4. During the rapprochement subphase, when the child may have tantrums and cry if the mother leaves for the evening, or for a few hours, or leaves the scene.

In all of these circumstances the child cannot tolerate visual or actual physical separation from the mother. Because of these conditions regarding separation, it is tempting to attribute separation problems and conflicts in adults to the time frame of the separation–individuation process in child development.

Dr. Frank's clinical study of his case is a model of psychoanalytic study and technique. I will refer first to his comment that the patient had a "problem with object constancy," which he believes "was associatively linked to her *anger and intensively ambivalent needs*" (my emphasis). The patient had insisted that if Dr. Frank were out of sight he was out of mind, and thus his psychological image changed with loss of the visual image. This particular passage is almost exactly paralleled by Mahler and colleagues' (1975) statement regarding one of the children Mahler had studied.

> As the third year of age progressed, Wendy began at times to protest actively, to cry vociferously, and to resist strongly her mother's departure from the room. She would still not be easily distracted from her sorrow.... She would withdraw and quietly sit on the little chair hugging a doll or a cuddly teddy bear.... At times, when Wendy felt so lonely and lost that she seemed almost paralyzed and out of contact, she appeared to lack the ability to retain an image of the mother, even though mother may have been in the adjoining room.... Thus, it seemed that momentarily she not only lacked emotional object constancy, but also that she lost its cognitive counterpart, Piaget's "mental image of the absent object." That is to say, she was not able to imagine where mother was when mother was not in her visual field. It seemed, at this time, that when mother was gone, there was not a "good mother image" intrapsychically available to Wendy. [p. 161]

Mahler speculated that this difficulty in object constancy had to do with Wendy's aggression and ambivalence; the mother described Wendy as a determined child who could, at times, get into battles with her at home and be quite negativistic. The similarity in the psychodynamic picture of Dr. Mahler's nursery child and Dr. Frank's adult patient is striking. Indeed, we are tempted to develop a reconstruction of early emotional life of Dr. Frank's patient and create another Wendy.

Early in the analysis (about the first six months) Dr. Frank indicated that his primary task was to avoid creating countertransference problems over issues concerning the couch. The patient had a problem lying on the couch, expressed concern about this, was not sure if she could trust the analyst, and spoke of her loneliness. At the same time, Dr. Frank was aware of the patient's need to provoke him and to replicate the relationship she reported with her father. If he either excused her from lying on the couch or verbally forced compliance with the traditional practice, "it would be suppressive and probably work against analysis, as well as be colluding in transferential acting out." Over the succeeding months, his hunch that the problem with the couch condensed important dynamic constellations was verified.

The question now is: What does all this have to do with the dynamics of the separation–individuation process? We can speculate that there are interesting parallels in the behavior of a 15- to 36-month-old child and the behavior and dynamics reported by Dr. Frank in his patient. For instance, during the rapprochement subphase, the child may constantly shadow the mother, keep her in visual contact, and incessantly ask questions whether answered or not; the substance of the replies are not as important as the fact that the mother listens and makes some response. Problems of insomnia in both children and adults (including Dr. Frank's patient) may relate to the difficulty in giving up the "object world," represented early in life by the mother. To isolate oneself from the "early mother" cannot be tolerated. In fact, it is dangerous, even if we invoke the Kleinian developmental idea of the "paranoid position," which presumably could make the presence of the mother dangerous if you can't "keep an eye" on her.

To lie on the analytic couch may stir up reminiscences of the danger of the recumbent position, the dangers of the object not being in sight; thus the vulnerability in lying down consists of losing sight of the object (mother). It may be that surrender and humiliation are also important factors, but they probably have little relationship to the early life of the child and would, from a developmental point of view, be more related to the oedipal or later phases of development.

In commenting on the problem the patient had in lying on the couch, Dr. Frank adds the following:

> If I was out of sight, I was out of mind; my psychological image changed with loss of my visual image. This problem with object constancy was associatively linked to her anger and intensely ambivalent needs. [p. 99]

Dr. Frank then deals more specifically with aspects of the rapprochement subphase of separation–individuation by the following description of the patient's behavior:

> The weekends played out the passions of the rapprochement phase, externally imposed by analytic scheduling. The internally motivated equivalent was demonstrable in her alternating self-contempt and resulting self-assertions over what she feared was passivity and neediness, and then angry provocative demands for the satisfactions they represented. [pp. 100–101]

In his subsequent discussion, the case material is presented as an unfolding drama highlighting the subphases of separation–individuation, vividly describing the intensity of the patient's reactions in the practicing and rapprochement phases of development; her ambivalence toward mother and father; her personal myths concerning father; the fusion of aggression with pre-oedipal and oedipal sexual striving and its manifestations in the transference; the issues involving strong sexual wishes and needs and its manifestations in the pre-oedipal and oedipal stages of development; and their impact on her relationships with a husband who is the multi-object on which her passive and active sexual wishes and behavior can be played out. Dr. Frank's descriptions are masterfully expressed in the technical language of a highly sophisticated and thoughtful analyst, interweaving a psychoanalytic fabric that encompasses the pre-oedipal (separation–individuation) and oedipal scenes as they can be seen today in the life of an educated, highly performing adult.

In the last portion of his chapter, Dr. Frank addresses the issue of separation and autonomy versus reengulfment and fusion during the termination phase. He describes these themes as they unfolded in the patient's productions and reactions. Again, the scenario involves elements of both the pre-oedipal and oedipal periods of life, as they "shaped" their way through latency, adolescence, and into adult life. With interesting ingenuity, Dr. Frank speaks of the "organizing theme of termination" as the patient initiated and planned the termination of the analysis. He writes: "My willingness to let her go, and her anticipation of my absence, signified rejection at each developmental level. She was the discarded forgotten baby, toddler, little boy and girl, school child, teenager and adult." In the drama of the last hour of the analysis, Dr. Frank describes the patient as tearful, experiencing the termination as the death of the analyst, and citing her anger for letting her go, in addition to losing him, but at the same time clearly recognizing the realities of the situation and expressing her gratitude and feeling of accomplishment. In a convincing style, he summarizes important features of the symptomatology as derivatives of the rapprochement subphase of development, and presents them in a style of a condensation or telescoping of developmental phases as they move through the developmental line, influencing and at the same time being impacted upon by the later oedipal, latency, adolescent, and adult life.

A significant statement by Dr. Frank embodies the thinking of Mahler, particularly her delineation of the stormy and character-forming phase of rapprochement. Dr. Frank says: "Of particular note was her [the patient's] use of the rapprochement phase as a template in the shaping and organizing of her emotional life as initially described and played out in the analysis." Following this, he comments on the confused and ambivalent feelings of gender identity, the inconstancy of identifications, the "problematic status of object constancy," and the internalization of a "savagely punitive superego." In a final statement, he emphasizes that all of the foregoing was largely initially acted in and acted out, experienced and represented, in the idiom of rapprochement as an organizational frame of reference.

Dr. Frank is an unusually gifted and creative writer of psychoanalysis. It is creative to formulate consensually accepted psychoanalytic theories, but even more creative to apply these theories to clinical phenomenology. The author has provided strong support for the idea that there are windows in the behavior and emotional life of the adult through which the behaviors and affect reactions of early childhood are visible, particularly in the 15- to 25-month-old child, when important aspects of the character and personality of the individual are formed. These qualities of the person modify and are modified along the lifeline of specific phase development, but core patterns developed during the separation–individuation phase of life can be recognized despite vicissitudes of development and the happenings of the external environment.

Dr. Frank has been very specific and correct in his use of the term "object constancy," but other writers have employed the term in ways that were not totally consonant with Mahler's use of the term. Perhaps a simplified way of understanding "object constancy" is to consider it as referring to a fixed, unchangeable internalized representation of mother as "a good mother" despite a multiplicity of variations in the theme of mother that occur in the course of the mother–child relationship, despite fights and accusations against her, or even threats of violence and attacks. The "good mother" is a core representation and, in my opinion, is essentially unchangeable from a dynamic standpoint. Object constancy, as a dynamic concept, should be differentiated from Piaget's (1936) "object permanence," a term applied to the cognitive retention of the memory of any object (human or not human) in its absence.

I have some reservations as to whether Dr. Frank's patient can be described as having a "developmental defect" in object constancy. Although there is evidence to suggest that there is a problem in object constancy, it may be that the internalized core representation of the mother is that of the good mother, which in the course of time has been "clouded" by defensive operations such as denial and projection in addition to other modifications. This "clouding" can seem to be a developmental defect, but we can attribute to it a quality of functional plasticity, unlike the "immutable" core representation of the good mother, which is not easily modifiable by analysis. It is this plasticity that permits the analytic process to modify and sometimes to bring to consciousness the good maternal object of constancy, which we might refer to as "the unforgettable and the unrememberable," quoting from Dr. Frank (1969) himself.

DR. MCLAUGHLIN'S CHAPTER

Dr. James T. McLaughlin discussed, in a delightful literary style (described by Dr. Sydney Pulver as lyrical, which I agree heartily), "kinetic patterns" of behavior, occurring not only during the sessions but also upon entry and departure from the analyst's office. Regardless of how we may feel about Dr. McLaughlin's interpretations of body movements, he brings to our attention the importance of including in the analyst's perceptions the slightest movement of the patient (even to the movement of fingers or deviation of gaze) and correlating this behavior with concurrent verbalizations by the patient. The charming reference by Dr. McLaughlin to the eyes-right-pass-in-review parades and the strange salute of the patient by quickly wiping of his nose and mouth with the back of his right hand as he passes the analyst on his way to the couch induces mental reverberations of army days in his own past that were not particularly pleasant for him. Perhaps a kind of folie à deux occurred between patient and analyst for a moment, both engaging in a mutual reciprocating salute that initiated the session, and continues as an entente à deux, usually referred to as the "psychoanalytic situation," in which the transference–countertransference is interlocked between patient and analyst in a continuing dyadic orbit, as the observer and the observed.

Dr. McLaughlin notes the precise gesticulations and hand movements and gaze of the patient while concurrently paying attention to the apparent affect and verbalizations of the patient, attempting from moment to moment to correlate bodily movements with specific constellations of thought and affect as revealed by the patient's verbalizations (a formidable task). Dr. McLaughlin comments on the contrast between off- and on-couch behavior in addition to other striking contrasts, such as movements and posture on the couch during the first year of the analysis as compared with later periods of the analysis.

Dr. McLaughlin notes a number of fascinating concurrences between the patient's verbal/affective associations and "specific kinesic patterning" when the patient was talking about his wife or other family members. At these times, the patient had no awareness of these correlations. For instance, when the patient talked of needing comfort or reassurance from his wife or sister, "the fingers of his left hand might free themselves to cover, and gently rub the back of his right hand." When speaking of his mother and commenting that he never knew whether she would be calm or assaultive, the kinesic linkage consisted of a thumb rapidly disappearing into the clasp of the other hand. The patient's mother also insisted upon obedience, sphincter control, and eating, and would become very angry if he did not comply or resisted her. However, he learned to capitulate to his mother for "fear of banishment," but became "stubborn and subversive," never capitulating completely.

As the analysis progressed and the patient became freer to express his controlled anger at his mother because of her constraints upon him, he would drum "on the back of one hand with the stiffened fingers of the other, back and forth, with great vigor and audible force," as he spoke of his helpless feelings to express himself for fear his mother would retaliate. This anxiety he feels to this day whenever he is subjected to anger from another person. Dr. McLaughlin notes that the finger drumming began to occur during silences in the analysis. He could then comment on the transference situation, especially the patient's need for reassurance and help from the analyst. In other words, the finger-drumming movement provided a clue to the patient's silence and a "window" in the transference situation at that moment.

Another type of kinesic movement, appearing toward the end of the first year of the analysis, consisted of an increase in tempo and prominence of thumb picking, to the point where occasional bleeding resulted. The increase was associated with the patient's ability to speak more fully of his needs and frustrations felt in relation to both parents and recently toward Dr. McLaughlin. The analyst now refers to a countertransference identification with the compulsive, bloody picking at the skin of both thumbs, prompting him to call attention for the first time in the analysis to this destructive habit, "partly out of mild concern for this self-mutilating, partly because I knew from my own analytic explorations of my own adolescent cuticle picking what rich dynamics of pent-up sexual conflict would lie in this behavior." Dr. McLaughlin also assumed that this picking was painful to the patient. The patient denied this and stated that he was unaware of his skin picking. He felt he would be given a beating and discharged by the analyst as being unanalyzable. Subsequently, though, the patient described his cuticle picking as a habit from early school years and was more forthright in speaking about it. He recalled his mother's "enraged screaming and face slapping" and the beatings by both parents. This led to the recalling of even earlier memories concerning thumb sucking and battles with his mother surrounding this habit, and subsequently to the acknowledgment of his lifelong struggle to stubbornly hold on to something that was his own, often at the cost of "mutuality and intimacy." Dr. McLaughlin states that in the subsequent course of treatment it was not necessary to address the hand kinesics directly.

Dr. McLaughlin summarizes his general thesis by commenting that the kinesic movements, or nonverbal components, may serve as metaphorical cues to underlying affective states and conflicts and support the analysts' understanding of the psychoanalytic situation from time to time. More specifically in relation to his first case, Dr. McLaughlin expresses some uncertainty as to the relevance of his clinical data to the issues of the separation–individuation process. I am inclined to agree with Dr. McLaughlin's concern at this point, because the symptom of nail and cuticle picking would more likely be a later development, that is, during the oedipal and latency periods. However, thumb sucking is quite common in infants and children prior to the oedipal phase of development. One certainly cannot exclude traumatic affective scenes occurring in the first three years of life (during separation–individuation) in relationship to thumb sucking as being an important precursor of characterological traits and personality development during the subsequent years of childhood, and there is no harm in speculating. I believe Dr. McLaughlin would be in agreement on this score. What is most impressive to me in this presentation is Dr. McLaughlin's masterful perceptions not only of the meaning and subtleties of the verbalizations of his patient, but also of their correlations with kinesic movements, not to mention the truly remarkable empathy he portrays in working with patients, enhanced certainly by constant attention to countertransference issues.

In describing his second case, Dr. McLaughlin exhibits more confidence in linking separation–individuation issues with his clinical data, particularly in relation to object constancy. The patient's nonverbal activity relates to her gaze of anxious vigilance, gut rumblings, restlessness on the couch, hand clutching, and twisting of a gold necklace. In addition, Dr. McLaughlin describes certain types of posturing (e.g., the "stirrup position") reminiscent of the times from the ages of 6 to 14 years when the patient was being treated for a chronic urinary tract problem and required frequent urological exams and procedures. Dr.

McLaughlin's ability to employ the kinesic cues assisted his own perceptual style of analytic listening (e.g., the "stirrup position" appearing at specific moments of the patient's preoccupations, or the "visual confrontations" employed by the patient on other occasions, all bearing a constellation of meanings referable to the patient's early relationship with mother, and now being reproduced in the transference). We should be grateful indeed to Dr. McLaughlin for noting this phenomenology in the analytic situation and bringing it to us with clarity and precision. His skilled management of both patients under conditions of stress and strong emotional reactions is the envy of all of us.

However, we must now evaluate the relevance of the current nonverbal behavior in the patients to the behavior in the separation–individuation process and determine whether we can peer through a current window and see the past as being reflected in the present. Here, I will quote a key statement from Dr. McLaughlin: "Both patients played out kinesically their oscillating between a reach for autonomy and separateness and their need for protected closeness." In his discussion, he clearly elaborates these oscillations in both of his patients, as enacted in their transference verbalizations and behaviors.

Dr. McLaughlin brings to our attention the advantages of kinesic cues presented by patients and reminds us that form and manner of communication, not just verbal content, provide insight into the preoccupations of the patient. Bodily positions, arm and hand movements, visual gaze, and the manner of entering and leaving the analyst's office may change in different ways during the course of the analysis. In his closing remark, Dr. McLaughlin emphasizes his conviction that "these kinesic and behavioral happenings do provide valuable cues to earlier struggles to individuate, and of longings for comforting closeness and reunion." But, he acknowledges his data to be a collage of circumstantial evidence and notes that there must be a point of which the advocate must rest his case. Dr. McLaughlin concludes, rather, poignantly, that consensual validation of sometimes lonely seekings need not lead to certainty, but is always a comfort. I strongly endorse these comments and hope that it provides some comfort (even though miniscule) to Dr. McLaughlin, who struggled so valiantly to demonstrate the reenactment of the subphases of separation–individuation in the analytic work, with references especially to the rapprochement subphase.

There is only one question I have that is a little troublesome to me, and that is that the father is almost totally absent in the report. There is increasing awareness that the father may play a more significant role in the separation–individuation process than previously thought, and Mahler (1980, personal communication) in her later years regretted that she had not studied the paternal input more adequately during her observations of the separation–individuation process. However, Dr. McLaughlin undoubtedly dealt with this issue during the analysis and preferred to report essentially the major issues involved.

CONCLUDING REMARKS

The essays contained in this book address one basic theme: the significance of the behavior and mental functioning in the child during the separation–individuation process for psychoanalytic theory and practice. The authors give us a considerable amount of information and data in a remarkable and fascinating manner. Nevertheless, a great deal of research is still needed to give a firmer scientific base to a consensus that so far has been derived from psychoanalytic treatment of a relatively few patients. At least two general areas must be explored in connection with the observations made by Mahler and her colleagues (1975) concerning the separation–individuation process in the young child: (a) its possible or potential impact upon the phallic-oedipal phase of development and the projections of this "mix" into subsequent periods of development into adulthood; and (b) the recognition of elements of this early behavior and mental functioning, or its derivatives, during the course of adult treatment, especially its use in reconstruction and technique.

Such research observations should be made by persons who have had dual-track training and experience—in research methodology and in psychoanalytic work. Fortunately, such "rare birds" are beginning to appear. (I might add that the American Psychoanalytic Association, in collaboration with the psychoanalytic section of the American Psychological Association, is actively sponsoring the development of such dual-track training.) One such rare bird is Dr. Robert N. Emde, who I am sure will forgive me for calling him such and who cautions that "we have probably placed far too much emphasis on early experience itself as opposed to the process by which it is modified or made use of by subsequent experience" (Emde 1981, p. 219). Also, regarding the resiliency in the infant, Emde says that we "probably need to tone down the attitude of irreversibility of adverse effects from early experience, even when it involves major deprivations of mothering. There is an urgent need to learn from case studies under psychoanalytic scrutiny" (p. 218).

I agree that psychoanalysts must employ a cautious brush in elaborating a full-grown adult psychodynamic landscape on an infant canvas or vice versa. However, there are times in psychoanalytic work when we can trace with some degree of confidence developmental continuities and personality configurations through the developmental lines without requiring extensive case histories of the past. At times, certain characteristics of personality, such as intense ambivalence in relation to parental figures, certain well-entrenched perversions, specific problems in gender identity, and other specific disturbances of drive or object preference may be traced through childhood and adolescence into adulthood. There is a risk, however, in excessive reconstruction work where, without much data of childhood and with little information regarding the family and its social milieu, a reconstruction of the separation–individuation phase of development is made by the analyst. What remains unquestioned, though, is that the concepts embodied in the work of Mahler and her colleagues represent a major advance in the understanding of early child development and in psychoanalytic practice and theory. These ideas have advanced our understanding of object-relations development and of the meaning of object constancy, and thereby the ideas of fusion, splitting, ambivalence, and ego boundaries. They have enriched our understanding of wide-ranging clinical phenomena such as narcissism, character neurosis, borderline personalities, and schizophrenia. Their impact on the technique of psychotherapy and psychoanalysis is to enlarge the scope of reconstruction and enhance the therapist's understanding of what the patient is truly unable to put into words.

REFERENCES

Balint, M. (1959). *Thrills and Regression.* London: Hogarth Press.
Bouvet, M. (1958). Technical variation and the concept of distance. *International Journal of Psycho-Analysis* 39:211-221.
Emde, R. N. (1981). Changing models of infancy and the nature of early development: remodeling the foundation. *Journal of the American Psychoanalytic Association* 29:179-219.
Frank, A. (1969). The unrememberable and the unforgettable: passive primal repression. *Psychoanalytic Study of the Child* 24:48-77. New York: International Universities Press.
Kris, E. (1956). The personal myth: a problem in psychoanalytic technique. *Journal of the American Psychoanalytic Association* 4:653-681.
Mahler, M. S. (1972). On the first three subphases of the separation-individuation process. In *The Selected Papers of Margaret S. Mahler,* vol. 2, pp. 119-130. New York: Jason Aronson, 1982.
Mahler, M. S., Pine, F., and Bergman, A. (1975). *The Psychological Birth of the Human Infant: Symbiosis and Individuation.* New York: Basic Books.
Pacella, B. L. (1980). The primal matrix configuration. In *Rapprochement: The Critical Subphase of Separation-Individuation,* ed. R. Lax, S. Bach, and A. Burland, pp. 117-131. New York: Jason Aronson.
Piaget, J. (1936). *The Origins of Intelligence in Children.* New York: International Universities Press, 1952.
Sandler, J. (1960). The background of safety. *International Journal of Psycho-Analysis* 41:352-360.
Spitz, R. A. (1965). *The First Year of Life.* New York: International Universities Press.
Weil, A. (1970). The basic core. *Psychoanalytic Study of the Child* 25:422-460. New York: International Universities Press.
Winnicott, D. W. (1958). The capacity to be alone. In *The Maturational Processes and the Facilitating Environment,* pp. 29-36. New York: International Universities Press.

Index

Abraham, K., 31
Adatto, C., 153
Agoraphobia, 31-32
  Deutsch on, 31
  Kohut on, 31
  Mittleman on, 31
  Roth on, 31
  Weiss on, 31
Akhtar, S.
  on negative therapeutic reaction, 51
  on optimal distance, immigration and, 45
  on self and object constancy, 9-10
  on separation-individuation, 11-12
  on severe personality disorders, 32-33
  on tether fantasy, 34
  immigration and, 44
Allport, G. W., 168
Ambitendency
  rapprochement and, 9
  tether fantasy and, 9
Anaclitic depression, 187

Analysis
  pre-oedipal issues in, 16
  preverbal issues in, 16
  visual images and, 36
Analytic process, optimal distance and, 82-84
Anthi, P., 154
Arlow, J. A., 100
  on nonverbal communication, 153
Asch, S.
  on depression and masochism, 119n
  on negative therapeutic reaction, 51

Bach, S., 23
Balint, M.
  on childhood games, 41
  on distance, 27-28, 184
  on ocnophilic attitude, 27-28
  on philobatic attitude, 27-28
  on physical contact, 62
  on tether fantasy, 68
Barnard, K., 62
Basic core, 181

Bathing habits, neurotic, 23
Beam, P., 71
Bergler, E., 123
Bergman, A.
  on mother–child distance, 29
  on tether fantasy and immigration, 44
Bernstein, S., 82
Birdwhistell, R. L., 168
Blos, P., 44
Blum, H., 32–33
Bodily ego, 4, 22
Boundaries, the oedipal barrier and, 66
Boundary sensitivity, 23
Bouvet, M.
  on distance, 24–25, 184
  on optimal distance, 62
    analytic, 50
    the couch and, 116
  on rapprochement, 25
Boyer, L. B., 48
Brazelton, T. B., 62
Burland, A. J., 34
Burlingham, D., 15
Burnham, H., 32–33

Cain, A. C., 11
Cain, B. S., 11
Campbell, R. J., 24
Child analysis
  Byerly on, 14
  countertransference and, 14–15
  difficulties of, 14
  informative alliance and, 15
  Kay on, 14
  Kramer on, 14
  Kris on, 15
  Mahler on, 13–14, 16–17
  nonverbal communication and, 13–14
  personal myth and, 15
  rescue fantasies and, 15
  theory and technique of, 13–17
  verbal intervention and, 14

Childhood games, optimal distance and, 41–42
Chmiel, A. J., 42–43
Cirlot, J. E., 40n
Claustrophobia, optimal distance and, 32
Communication
  explicit, 2
  nonverbal, 2
Cooper, A.
  on analytic process, 82
  on masochism, 123–124
  on optimal distance, 82
  on pain and separation-individuation, 127
Corney, R. T., 39
Couch, the
  optimal distance and, 116
  problems with
    clinical presentation, 94–109
    Fenichel on, 91
    Freud, S. on, 91
    Glover on, 91
    Greenson on, 92
    Hartmann on, 117
    lying down, meaning of, 116–118
    McAloon on, 92
    Montagnier on, 91–92
    object constancy and, 118–119
    Orens on, 92
    Reiser on, 93
    Roazen on, 116
    Silber on, 93
    Spitz on, 91
    Weissman on, 93
    Winnicott on, 93
Countertransference
  child analysis and, 14–15
  Jacobs on, 84
  optimal distance and, 84

Depressive masochistic personality, 119, 122–123
Deutsch, F.
  on posturology, 23

Index 203

on nonverbal communication, 153, 168
Deutsch, H., on agoraphobia, 31, 32–33
Developmental deficit, 187
Dewall, 43
Differentiation, 5–6
Distance. *See also* Optimal distance
  Balint on, 27–28, 184
  Bergman on, 29
  Bouvet on, 24–25, 184
  gender differences and, 29n
  incest barrier and, 34n
  Mahler on, 29n
  mother–child, 29, 29n
  oedipal phase and, 34
  perception, 28
  Spitz on, 28, 184
  Winnicott on, 29n
Distance, the concept of
  negative therapeutic reaction and, 50
  tact and, 46
  technical implications and, 46–52
  usage of, 23–26
Dual-track training, 199
Dunlap, K., 168

Edward, J., 9, 63
Ego boundary formation, 185
Eissler, K., 152
Emblem, definition of, 172–173
Emde, R. N., 199
Erikson, E.,
  on identity fusion, 62
  on optimal distance, games and, 41
Escoll, P. 82

Fairbairn, W. R. D., 33
Fenichel, O.
  on bathing habits, 23
  on distance, 24
  on problems with the couch, 91
Ferenczi, S. 152

Feyereisen, P., 170–171
Fine, B. D., 24
Fischer, N., 40, 67
Fraiberg, S., 107
Frank, A.
  on object constancy, 100
  on preverbal expression, 121
  on preverbal trauma, 16n
  on reconstruction, 120
  on tether fantasy, 34
Freud, A.
  on object constancy, 100
  on optimal distance, 50, 83
Freud, S.
  on bodily ego, 4, 22
  on body and intrapsychic processes, 11
  on bungled actions, 23
  on distance, 23n
  on falling in love, 35
  on frustrating experiences, 5
  on fundamental rule of analysis, 114
  on instinctual renunciation, 33
  on mind–body connection, 61
  on negative therapeutic reaction, 50
  on nonverbal communication, 132, 152, 168
  on optimal distance, games and, 41
  on psychic pain, immigration and, 44
  on repressed prostitution fantasy, 31
  on resistance to the couch, 91
  and tether fantasy, 40
Frustrating experiences
  Freud, S. on, 5
  Jacobson on, 4–5
  Kramer on, 4–5
  role of in psychic development, 4–5

Galenson, E.
  on the pre-oedipal genital phase, 104
  on rapprochement, 126
Gediman, H. K., 33

Gesture
    definition of, 170
    Feyereisen on, 170–171
    McNeill on, 170–171
    Walzer on, 170–171
Gibran, K., 32
Gill, M., 84
Gilligan, C., 63
Glenn, G., 41–42
Glover, E.
    on floating tranferences, 125
    on problems with the couch, 91
Gould, R., 65
Greenacre, P.
    on nonverbal communication, 2
    on Oedipus complex, 16
    on reconstruction, 120
    on separation experiences, 28n
Greenson, R.
    on gender differences in
        rapprochement, 8
    on problems with the couch, 92
    on transference, 125
Grindberg, L. R., 44, 45
Grinstein, A., 43
Groddeck, G., 152, 168
Gruenert, U., 51
Gunderson, J., 32–33
Guntrip, H.,
    on optimal distance, analysis and, 48
    on separation-individuation, 62
    on severe personality disorders, 33
Guttman, S. A., 23n

Handelman, S., 75
Hartman, H., 117
Herman, J., 124
Hinsie, L. E., 24
Hoffer, W.
    on masochism, 123
    on silent trauma, 121–122
    on touch, importance of, 5n
Hoffman, I. Z., 165
Hollander, M., 62
Horowitz, L.
    on nonverbal communication, 152
    on optimal distance, 82

Identity fusion, 62
Inability to sleep
    Fraiberg on, 107
    La Perriere on, 107–108
    Mahler on, 107–108
Incest barrier, 34n
Informative alliance, 15

Jacobs, T.
    on countertransference, 84
    on nonverbal communication, 154
Jacobson, E., 4–5
James, W. T., 168
Jones, R. L., 23n

Kaplan, 43n
Kay, P., 14, 16
Kegan, R., 64
Kernberg, O. F.
    on depression and masochism, 119n
    on depressive personality, 122–123
    on masochistic personality, 119
    on severe personality disorders,
        32–33
Kestenberg, J. S., 127
Kinesics
    Allport on, 168
    Birdwhistell on, 168
    Dunlap on, 168
    enactments and, 165–169
    hand-snout, 153
    James on, 168
    Krout on, 168
    Scheflen on, 168
    Vernon on, 168
    Wolff on, 168
Klauber, J., 46
Kleeman, J. A., 41–42
Kohut, H., 31
Kramer, S.
    on frustrating experiences, 5

Index

on object constancy, 118
on self and object constancy, 9–10
on separation-individuation, 11–12
Kris, E.
   on child analysis, 15
   on personal myth, 96, 120, 180
   on strain trauma, 121
Krout, M. H., 168

La Perriere, K., 107–108
Laplanche, J., 24
Lax, E., 67
Lebovici, S., 11
Lester, S., 121
Levine, H., 82
Lilleskov, R., 154
Locomotor anxiety, 31
Loewald, H., 120
   on the ego, 121
   on Oedipus complex, 11
   on optimal distance, 83
   on separation, 128
   on vulva dread, 126
Loewenstein, R.
   on distance, interpretations and, 83
   on optimal distance, tact and, 50

McAloon, R., 92
McDevitt, J., 4
McLaughlin, J. T.
   on nonverbal communication, 154
   on observing and note taking, 134
   on transference, 17
   on transference-countertransference, 165
McNeill, D.
   on emblems, 170
   on gestures, 170–171
Mahler, M. S.
   on child analysis techniques, 16–17
   on childhood games and, 41
   on differentiation, 29

on ego boundary formation, 185
on emotional object constancy, 188
on gender differences
   and distance, 29n
   in rapprochement, 8
on inability to sleep, 107–108
on nonverbal communication 13–14
on object constancy, 100, 118
on Oedipus complex, 11
on optimal distance, 25–27
on penis envy, 126
on rapprochement, 7, 105
   crisis in, 28–29
on separation-individuation
   optimal distance and, 62
   paternal input and, 198
   phallic-oedipal phase and, 198
   process, 181
on somatic inputs, significance of, 4
on symbiosis
   and individuation, 180
   mother-child, 3
on symbiotic orbit, 39
on symbiotic and practicing phases, 28
on tactile sensations, 62
on tether fantasy, 34, 39
Masochism
   Bergler on, 123
   Cooper on, 123, 124
   Herman on, 124
   Hoffer on, 123
   separation-individuation and, 122–124
Melges, F. T., 32–33
Miller, J., 51n
Mittleman, B., 31
Modell, A., 51
Montagnier, M. T., 91–92
Moore, B. E., 24
Multiple function
   Waelder on, 63
   principle of, 34

Needles, W., 153
Negative therapeutic reaction, 50
  Akhtar on, 51
  Asch on, 51
  Gruenert on, 51
  Miller on, 51n
  Modell on, 51
Nonverbal behavior
  emblems, 170
  gestures, 170
  McNeill on, 170
  modes of, 169–174
  technical implications of, 174–175
Nonverbal communication
  Adatto, on, 153
  Anthi on, 155
  Arlow on, 153–154
  clinical examples, 132–151
  Deutsch on, 153, 168
  Ferenczi on, 152
  Freud, S. on, 132, 152, 168
  Groddeck on, 152, 168
  Jacobs on, 155
  Lilleskov on, 154
  McLaughlin on, 154, 155
  Mushatt on, 155
  Needles on, 153
  Noy on, 154
  Rangell on, 153
  Sacks on, 154
  Shapiro on, 155
  Suslick on, 153
Noy, P., 154

Object constancy, 118–119
  Frank on, 100
  Freud, A. on, 100
  Kramer on, 118
  Mahler on, 100, 118, 188
  separation-individuation and, 62
Object permanence, 100, 192
Ocnophilic attitude, 27–28
Oedipal phase, distance and, 34

Oedipus complex
  Lebovici on, 11
  Loewald on, 11
  Mahler on, 11
Optimal closeness, 63
Optimal distance
  agoraphobia and, 31
  the analytic process and, 82–84
    Bernstein on, 82
    Cooper on, 82
    Escoll on, 82
    Freud, A., on, 83
    Horwitz on, 82
    Levine on, 82
  animal behavior and, 69–73
  Balint on, 41, 62
  Beam on, 71
  boundaries and, 66
  Bouvet on, 62
  childhood games and, 41–42
  claustrophobia and, 32
  clinical illustration, 76–82
  concept of, 61–65
  definitions of, 23–26
  developmental perspective of, 26–31
  Erikson on, 41
  fiction and, 74–76
  Freud on, 41
  Glenn on, 41–42
  Gould on, 65
  Handelman on, 75
  homesickness and, 65
  immigration and
    Akhtar on, 45
    Blos on, 44
    Dewall on, 43
    Teja on, 45
  interpretations and
    Gill and, 84
    Loewald and, 83
    Loewenstein and, 83
  Kleeman on, 41–42
  Lax on, 67

Index 207

Loewenstein on, 50
Mahler on, 25–27, 41
marriage and
   Barnes on, 32
   Gibran on, 32
mother and child and, 25–27
painting and, 71–73
parenting and, 64
Phillips on, 41
physical contact and, 62
poetry and, 76
Poland on, 50
Prown on, 71
psychic position and, 30
psychopathology of, 31–33
psychotherapist–patient and
   Bouvet on, 50
   Boyer on, 48
   Freud, A. on, 50
   Guntrip on, 48
   Strachey on, 50
   Volkan on, 48
   Winnicott on, 49
Schopenhauer on, 31
sculpture and, 73–74
separation-individuation and, 63
severe personality disorders and, 32–33
sexuality and aggression and, 65–67
sociocultural vicissitude and, 41–46
Stewart on, 62
tact and, 50
tactile sensations and, 62
tether fantasy and, 67–69
travel and
   Balint on, 42–43
   Chmiel on, 42
   Grinstein on, 43
   Kaplan on, 43n
   Waelder on, 41
   Winnicott on, 41
Orens, M., 92

Pacella, B. L., 181–182
Parens, H., 6
Parenting, gender differences and, 63
Parrish, 23n
Penis envy, 126
Personal myth
   child analysis and, 15
   Kris on, 96, 120, 180
Personality disorders
   Akhtar on, 32–33
   Blum on, 32
   Burnham on, 32–33
   Deutsch, H. on, 32–33
   Fairbairn on, 33
   Gediman on, 33
   Gunderson on, 32–33
   Guntrip on, 33
   Kernberg on, 32–33
   Melges on, 32–33
   optimal distance and, 32–33
   Swartz on, 32–33
Phallic-oedipal phase, 11
Philbatic attitude, 27–28
Phillips, R. H., 41
Piaget, J., 100, 192
Pine, F., 173
Poland, W. S.
   on the incest barrier, 34n
   on optimal distance, tact and, 50
   on tact, 46
Pollock, G., 44
Pontalis, J. B., 24
Postural oddities, 23
Poznanski, E. O., 11
Pre-oedipal genital phase
   Galenson and Roiphe on, 104
   rapprochement and, 104
Preverbal
   expression, 121
   trauma, 16n
Proprioenteroceptive experiences, 4
Prown, J., 71
Pruett, K., 63

Psychic pain
  Freud S., on, 44
  immigration and, 44
Psychotherapist, the, tact and
  Klauber on, 46
  Poland on, 46

Rangell, L., 153
Rapprochement
  ambitendency and, 9
  cognitive strides in, 9
  crisis, 28–29
  definition of, 25
  Galenson on, 126
  gender differences in, 8
  Greenson on, 8
  intrapsychic developments in, 7–8
  Mahler on, 7, 8, 28–29, 105
  the phallic-oedipal phase and, 11
  the pre-oedipal genital phase and, 104
  Roiphe on, 126
  separation-individuation and, 30, 7–9
  Settlage on, 7
  tether fantasy and, 34
  Tolpin on, 7
Reconstruction
  early trauma and, 119–122
  Frank on, 120
  Greenacre on, 120
  Valenstein on, 120
Reiser, L., 93
Replacement child, the, 11
Repressed prostitution fantasy, 31
Rescue fantasies, child analysis and, 15
Riess, A., 4
Ritvo, S., 11
Roazen, P., 116
Roiphe, H., 126
Role responsiveness, 126
Rosenfeld, H. A., 125

Rossner, J., 23
Roth, M., 31
Rubinfine, D., 121
Ruskin, N., 9
Rycroft, C., 24

Sacks, O., 154
Sandler, J., 182
  on role responsiveness, 126
  on screen trauma, 121
Scheflen, A. E., 168
Schopenhauer, A., 31
Schwaber, E., 84
  on transference-countertransference, 165
Screen
  dream, 181
  trauma, 121
  waking, 181–182
Searles, H., 125
Self and object constancy, 11
Sensoriperceptive experiences, 4
Separation, 128
  experiences, 28n
Separation-individuation
  Akhtar on, 9–10
  ambitendency and, 30
  clinical illustration of, 11–13
  Cooper on, 127
  differentiation phase in, 29
  Furer on, 6
  Guntrip on, 62
  Kestenberg on, 127
  Kramer on, 9–10
  Mahler on, 62, 173, 181, 198
  masochism and, 122–124
  object constancy and, 62
  optimal distance, 62–63
  pain and, 127
  paternal input and, 198
  periods of, 187
  phallic-oedipal phase and, 198
  Pine on, 173
  practicing, 6–7

Index   209

Parens on, 6
and rapprochement, 7–9
    subphase in, 30
and self and object constancy, 9–11
Shapiro, T., 154
Silber, A., 93
Silent trauma, 121–122
Somatic inputs, 4
Spitz, R.
    on anaclitic depression, 187
    on distance, 184
    on distance perception, 28
    on problems with couch, 91
Sterba, E., 44
Stewart, H., 62
Strachey, J., 50
Strain trauma, 121
Suslick, A., 153
Swartz, M. S., 32–33
Symbiosis
    individuation and, 180
    Mahler on, 3, 180
    mother-child, 3
    review of, 3–5
Symbiotic
    bonds, Winnicott on, 127–128
    orbit, Mahler on, 39
    phase, Weil on, 3–4, 122
    and practicing phases, Mahler on, 28

Tactile sensations
    Brazelton on, 62
    Hollander on, 62
    importance of, 62
    optimal distance and, 62
Teja, J. S., 45
Tether fantasy, 33–41, 67–69
    Akhtar on, 34
    ambitendency and, 9
    Balint on, 68
    Burland on, 34
    Cirlot on, 40n
    clinical cases, 35–38

Corney on, 39
distance contact and, 39
Edward on, 9
Fischer and, 40, 67
Frank on, 34
Freud, S. and, 40
immigration and
    Akhtar on, 44
    Bergman on, 44
    Grindberg on, 44, 45
instinctual renunciation and, 33
Mahler on, 34, 39
Pollock on, 44
rapprochement and, 34
Ruskin on, 9
symbiotic orbit and, 39
telephone and, 68
Turrini on, 9
Volkan on, 39
Winnicott and, 40
Touch, importance of, 5n
Transference-countertransference
    Greenson on, 125
    Schwaber on, 165
Transferences
    archaic, 124–127
    floating, 125
    McLaughlin on, 165
Transitional objects
    Rosenfeld on, 125
    Searles on, 125
    Winnicott on, 44
Transitional phenomena, 158
Trauma, silent, 121–122
Turrini, P., 9

Unexplained nausea, 23

Valenstein, A., 120
Verbal intervention in child analysis, 14
Vernon, P. E., 168
Visual images, analysis and, 36

Volkan, V. D.
  on optimal distance, 48
  on tether fantasy, 39
Vulva dread, 126

Waelder, R.
  on multiple function, principle of, 34, 63
  on optimal distance, 41
Walzer, D., 170–171
Weil, A., 3, 122, 181
Weissman, S., 93

Winnicott, D.
  on development deficit, 187
  on mother–child distance, 29n
  on optimal distance, 41, 49
  on problems with couch, 93
  on symbiotic bonds, 127–128
  and tether fantasy, 40
  on transitional objects, 44
  on transitional phenomena, 158
Wolff, C., 168

Zeligs, M., 153